Enhancing Cognitive Functioning and Brain Plasticity

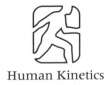

Human Kinetics

Aging, Exercise, and Cognition Series

VOLUME 3

Leonard W. Poon, PhD

Waneen W. Spirduso, EdD

Wojtek Chodzko-Zajko, PhD

SERIES EDITORS

Enhancing Cognitive Functioning and Brain Plasticity

Wojtek Chodzko-Zajko, PhD
University of Illinois at Urbana-Champaign

Arthur F. Kramer, PhD
University of Illinois at Urbana-Champaign

Leonard W. Poon, PhD
University of Georgia

EDITORS

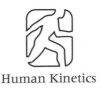

Human Kinetics

Library of Congress Cataloging-in-Publication Data

Enhancing cognitive functioning and brain plasticity / Wojtek Chodzko-Zajko,
Arthur F. Kramer, Leonard W. Poon, editors.
    p. ; cm. -- (Aging, exercise, and cognition series ; v. 3)
    Includes bibliographical references and index.
    ISBN-13: 978-0-7360-5791-2 (hard cover)
    ISBN-10: 0-7360-5791-9 (hard cover)
    1. Cognition--Effect of exercise on. 2. Exercise--Psychological aspects. 3.
Neuroplasticity. 4. Cognition in old age. I. Chodzko-Zajko, Wojtek J. II.
Kramer, Arthur F. III. Poon, Leonard W., 1942- IV. Series: Aging, exercise,
and cognition series ; v. 3.
    [DNLM: 1. Aging--physiology. 2. Cognition--physiology. 3. Aged. 4.
Brain--physiology. 5. Exercise. 6. Neuronal Plasticity--physiology. WT 145
E58 2009]
    BF311.E54 2009
    155.67'13--dc22

                                   2009013298

ISBN-10: 0-7360-5791-9 (print)   ISBN-10: 0-7360-8542-4 (Adobe PDF)
ISBN-13: 978-0-7360-5791-2 (print)   ISBN-13: 978-0-7360-8542-7 (Adobe PDF)

Acquisitions Editor: Judy Patterson Wright, PhD; **Managing Editor:** Lee Alexander;
Copyeditor: Joyce Sexton; **Proofreader:** Kathy Bennett; **Indexer:** Joan K. Griffitts; **Permission Manager:** Dalene Reeder; **Graphic Designer:** Nancy Rasmus; **Graphic Artist:**
Dawn Sills; **Cover Designer:** Bob Ruether; **Art Manager:** Kelly Hendren; **Associate Art
Manager:** Alan L. Wilborn; **Illustrator:** Alan L. Wilborn; **Printer:** Thomson-Shore, Inc.

Printed in the United States of America   10 9 8 7 6 5 4 3 2 1

The paper in this book is certified under a sustainable forestry program.

Human Kinetics
Web site: www.HumanKinetics.com

United States: Human Kinetics
P.O. Box 5076
Champaign, IL 61825-5076
800-747-4457
e-mail: humank@hkusa.com

Canada: Human Kinetics
475 Devonshire Road Unit 100
Windsor, ON N8Y 2L5
800-465-7301 (in Canada only)
e-mail: info@hkcanada.com

Europe: Human Kinetics
107 Bradford Road
Stanningley
Leeds LS28 6AT, United Kingdom
+44 (0) 113 255 5665
e-mail: hk@hkeurope.com

Australia: Human Kinetics
57A Price Avenue
Lower Mitcham, South Australia 5062
08 8372 0999
e-mail: info@hkaustralia.com

New Zealand: Human Kinetics
Division of Sports Distributors NZ Ltd.
P.O. Box 300 226 Albany
North Shore City
Auckland
0064 9 448 1207
e-mail: info@humankinetics.co.nz

CONTENTS

Contents

CONTRIBUTORS

Brenda J. Anderson, PhD
Department of Psychology and the Program in Neuroscience, SUNY Stony Brook

Sarah M. Buck
Department of Health, Physical Education, and Recreation, Chicago State University

Kirk I. Erickson, PhD
Department of Psychology, University of Illinois at Urbana-Champaign

Jennifer L. Etnier, PhD
Department of Exercise and Sport Science, University of North Carolina at Greensboro

Monica Fabiani
Beckman Institute and Psychology Department, University of Illinois at Urbana-Champaign

Gabriele Gratton
Beckman Institute and Psychology Department, University of Illinois at Urbana-Champaign

Charles H. Hillman, PhD
Department of Kinesiology and Community Health, University of Illinois at Urbana-Champaign

Keita Kamijo, PhD
Institute for Human Science and Biomedical Engineering, National Institute of Advanced Industrial Science and Technology

Donna L. Korol
Department of Psychology, University of Illinois at Urbana-Champaign

Daniel P. McCloskey
Department of Psychology, City University of New York, Staten Island

Michelle L. Meade
Department of Psychology, Montana State University

Nefta A. Mitchell
Department of Psychology, SUNY Stony Brook

Daniel G. Morrow
Institute of Aviation, University of Illinois at Urbana-Champaign

Denise C. Park, PhD
School of Behavioral and Brain Sciences, University of Texas at Dallas

Carmi Schooler, PhD
National Institutes of Health, Department of Health and Human Services

Despina A. Tata
Department of Psychology, Aristotle University of Thessaloniki

Jason R. Themanson
Department of Psychology, Illinois Wesleyan University

PREFACE

This volume is the third of a series of edited books that examine the complex role of exercise and physical activity in cognitive functioning of older adults from a variety of perspectives. The first volume in the series provided a review of exercise and cognition issues in general and summarized information about the physiological mechanisms relevant to the understanding of cognitive changes that occur among older adults (Poon, Chodzko-Zajko, & Tomporowski, 2006). The second volume addressed mediating and moderating processes that produce individual variations in the impact of exercise on cognition (Spirduso, Poon, & Chodzko-Zajko, 2007). This third and final volume deals with both exercise and nonexercise interventions that have been shown to influence cognitive and brain plasticity in older human and nonhuman animals. In all three volumes, researchers and practitioners who are skilled in exercise, cognition, aging, neurological or biological mechanisms, or more than one of these areas came together to discuss these processes and then wrote chapters for the volumes. It is interesting to note that few authors are experts in all domains, and the goals of the chapters are to encourage synergy in addressing the complex issues involved in exercise, physical activities, and cognition in old age.

In Volume Three, the first chapter by Fabiani and Gratton sets the stage for later chapters by briefly describing theories of cognitive aging that have, for the most part, been developed on the basis of behavioral data. The authors then describe how a variety of complementary neuroimaging measures, including event-related brain potentials, positron emission tomography, functional magnetic resonance imaging, and event-related optical imaging, have been used to both test and extend theories of cognitive aging. They also focus on how these neuroimaging measures have been used to study individual differences in cognition and brain function particularly with regard to adult aging. They conclude with a prescription for future research that focuses on the study of adult aging from both psychological and neuroscience perspectives.

The next three chapters focus on the influence of cognitive training, intellectual engagement (including cognitively complex work and leisure activities), and expertise effects on the improvement and maintenance of selective and general aspects of cognition throughout adulthood. In the second chapter, Carmi Schooler examines the potential reciprocal relationships between paid employment and leisure-time activities and intellectual functioning among older adults. His chapter provides compelling evidence that continuing to perform intellectually demanding activities in mid and later life, during both paid employment and leisure-time activities, is associated with positive cognitive and psychosocial outcomes. Interestingly, there is also a modest reciprocal relationship such that intellectual functioning influences the cognitive complexity of work and leisure-time activities to which individuals are exposed. Schooler argues that examining the cognitive effects of occupational and nonoccupational activities is of direct interest to those concerned with understanding how the environment affects the psychological functioning of older people.

Next, Meade and Park examine the impact of several nonexercise interventions on human cognitive functioning in older adults. Specifically, their chapter provides a comparison of the effectiveness of highly controlled laboratory interventions, in which subjects are trained in an effort to improve specific cognitive functions, and a variety of more realistic lifestyle interventions that have been shown to assist in the preservation of cognitive functioning in older adults. Meade and Park argue that although most cognitive training studies focus on improving effortful cognitive processes, with which older adults have difficulty, a complementary strategy is to capitalize on cognitive processes that are relatively age invariant (i.e., performed relatively automatically) as a means to enhance overall cognitive function. They provide a compelling example of how this might be achieved from the arena of medical monitoring. Lifestyle factors, including social interaction, are also discussed in terms of their influence on cognitive function in adulthood.

In chapter 4, the final chapter in this section, Morrow examines the literature that has addressed the relationship between expertise and aging. More specifically, his critical review examines how, and to what extent, expertise in a particular work, sport, or leisure context reduces age-related declines in both context-specific skills and broader cognitive processes and abilities. Morrow comes to the conclusion that the maintenance of high levels of skill requires deliberate and continued practice in a domain as well as the development of knowledge-based strategies. Furthermore, maintenance of high levels of skills during aging depends on the characteristics of the person, the task, and the manner in which performance is assessed. Finally, expertise effects tend to be relatively narrow and pertain mostly to the domain in which expertise is acquired rather than to general cognitive abilities.

The next four chapters focus on the influence of specific interventions on performance, cognition, and brain function of older organisms in both human and nonhuman models. In chapter 5, Anderson, McCloskey, Mitchell, and Tata provide a detailed review of what we currently know about exercise training effects, with nonhuman animals, on a variety of brain regions including the hippocampus, cerebellum, motor cortex, and striatum. The authors examine the extent to which exercise training effects on performance, learning, and memory are a consequence of the selective effects of exercise on specific neural systems and mechanisms or an indirect consequence of general hormonal and vascular responses to exercise. Their review suggests that exercise has selective effects on brain areas and that these effects are implicated in the mediation of cognitive improvements in aging, as reflected in changes in learning and memory. In chapter 6, Hillman, Buck, and Themanson review the experimental literature pertaining to the role of exercise and physical activity in aspects of neurocognitive functioning across the life span. The authors argue that there is now a wealth of evidence that lifestyle factors protect against cognitive loss during aging. They review the literature suggesting that aging is associated with disproportionate decrements in executive control processes relative to other types of cognition and that these declines can be reduced by exercise interventions. In particular, they summarize evidence for an association between exercise and physical activity and event-related brain potential (ERP) activity.

In chapter 7, Keita Kamijo examines issues related to the measurement and assessment of the acute effects of physical activity on several indices of neuroelectric functioning. Kamijo provides an overview of the relationship between acute exercise and ERPs. The chapter reviews methodological issues related to the measurement of various components of the ERP in exercise studies, examining not only the P3 wave but also several earlier stimulus-locked components (e.g., N1, P2, and N2), as well as the contingent negative variation (CNV) and error-related negativity (ERN). The chapter concludes with a discussion of the effects of acute exercise on ERP indices of cognitive processing in older adults. In the last chapter in this section, Erickson and Korol examine the impact of a widely employed nonexercise intervention, hormone replacement therapy (HRT), on cognitive performance in older women. Specifically, they review and synthesize neuroimaging research, on both brain structure and brain function, that addresses the effects of HRT in postmenopausal women. On the basis of findings from preclinical and clinical studies, they argue that HRT affects the brains of postmenopausal women in a complex and multifactorial fashion, targeting some brain areas and neural mechanisms but not others. The authors suggest that future work should utilize neuroimaging techniques to assess the impact of hormone therapy on cognitive and brain health in women.

The final chapter considers implications of research on aging, exercise, and cognition for public health and public policy recommendations. Jennifer Etnier considers whether the strength of the evidence underlying the relationship between exercise and physical activity interventions and cognitive improvement is sufficient to support specific public health recommendations. Etnier concludes that based on available evidence, the prescription of physical activity for the protection or improvement of cognitive performance is warranted. However, she cautions that specific details regarding the optimal exercise prescription have yet to be clarified. Additional research is needed before specific recommendations can be made regarding the exact type, intensity, and frequency of physical activity needed to enhance cognitive performance in older adults.

The third Exercise, Cognition, and Aging workshop was sponsored by the University of Illinois' Initiative on Aging, the College of Applied Health Sciences, the NIH Center for Healthy Minds, the Beckman Institute, and the National Blueprint Office at the University of Illinois at Urbana-Champaign. The workshop was held at the Levis Faculty Center, Urbana, Illinois, on October 19-20, 2004. We acknowledge the valuable assistance and participation of Lisa Sheppard, Deb Shilts, and Chae-Hee Park, whose efforts made the conference and this volume possible.

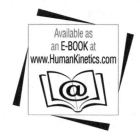

Available as
an E-BOOK at
www.HumanKinetics.com

CHAPTER 1

Brain Imaging Probes Into the Cognitive and Physiological Effects of Aging

Monica Fabiani

Beckman Institute and Psychology Department,
University of Illinois at Urbana-Champaign

Gabriele Gratton

Beckman Institute and Psychology Department,
University of Illinois at Urbana-Champaign

Cognitive aging is both a very important practical concern and a health-related problem because it influences (directly or indirectly) a large proportion of the U.S. population. Therefore, not surprisingly, it is the target of a large number of studies in a variety of domains—from basic science work to applied work in the fields of gerontology and geriatrics. In this chapter we present a selective review of psychophysiological and brain imaging data. We highlight possible mechanisms that may underlie cognitive aging in the context of extant psychological theories of aging based on behavioral data. We also emphasize the role of individual differences in enhancing our understanding of the main factors underlying age-related changes.

Theories of Cognitive Aging: Behavioral, Psychophysiological, and Neuroimaging Evidence

Normal cognitive aging is characterized mainly by problems of memory, attention, and easy fatigue, whereas language abilities appear relatively spared (Park et al., 1996). Psychologists have developed three major theories to account for the effects of cognitive aging. These accounts, which are not necessarily mutually exclusive, include (a) generalized slowing

This work was supported by ADRD grant #C-6-29710 and NIA grant #AG21887 to Monica Fabiani.

(Salthouse, 1996; for a review see Birren & Fisher, 1995), (b) diminished inhibitory processes (Hasher & Zacks, 1988), and (c) deficits in working memory function (Craik & Byrd, 1982). These theories are largely based on behavioral outcomes obtained from comparison of younger and older adults' performance in cognitive tasks, and are briefly reviewed later in this section. In the last 15 years, the increased availability of noninvasive imaging tools has made it possible to start investigating the physiological and anatomical bases of cognitive aging. This knowledge promises to be extremely useful in identifying target areas that may be amenable to intervention—in the form of either preventive action or remediation.

Generalized Slowing of Cognitive Processes

Slowing of cognitive processing is typically observed in normal aging using reaction time or other speeded tasks (Salthouse, 1996). Birren and Fisher (1995) review an extensive series of studies and conclude that almost all tasks in which speed is a factor are impaired in aging. Basic measures of electroencephalographic rhythms (such as the alpha rhythm) are reported to be slowed down in aging (for a review see Woodruff-Pak, 1997). Similarly, psychophysiological measures of the latency of brain responses (such as the latency of the P300 component of the event-related brain potential, ERP) show clear latency increases with aging (Polich et al., 1985).

Reduced Inhibitory Function

Hasher and Zacks (1988) observed that older adults have more difficulty than younger adults in inhibiting prepotent responses that are no longer appropriate. Further they observed that tasks involving response conflict are disproportionately affected by aging. Finally, evidence indicates that older adults are more easily distracted by irrelevant stimuli than younger subjects (Kausler & Hakami, 1982; see also Rabbitt, 1965). Taken together, these data suggest a reduced ability of older adults to inhibit processes or responses that are not directly relevant to the task at hand. Psychophysiological and neuroimaging evidence consistent with this view is reviewed later in this section.

Deficits in Working Memory

Several authors have observed that aging is associated with a decline of executive and working memory function (West, 1996; Moscovitch & Winocur, 1992). In several cases, the working memory deficits are most evident when distracters are used during the test. These and other similar data point to a strong relationship between working memory and attention control (e.g., Kane & Engle, 2000). In this context, the reduced-inhibition account just discussed can also explain the working memory deficit often observed in older adults (as a reflection of interference effects, e.g., Bowles & Salthouse, 2003). It is also possible to use the reduced-inhibition hypothesis to account for generalized slowing effects, as the latter can be the result of more "noise" at multiple levels within the information-processing system.

Psychophysiological Evidence

Research on cognitive aging based on ERP measures has yielded substantial evidence in favor of both slowing of processes and reduced inhibition. The first phenomenon is typically demonstrated by increases in the latency of various ERP components as a function of age (Polich et al., 1985). For instance, the latency of P300 increases by about 1 or 2 ms per year (on average) between the ages of 20 and 80 years (Polich et al., 1985). Age-related increases in P300 latency, however, are often dissociated from the corresponding increases in reaction time (Smulders et al., 1999). Because P300 latency is often considered sensitive to stimulus evaluation time and relatively less influenced by response processes (see Fabiani et al., 2007), these data suggest that both stimulus evaluation and response processes are delayed in aging, consistent with the generalized slowing hypothesis. However, there are also cases in which effects of age on ERP latency appear more specific to particular intervals, and thus perhaps attributable to specific processing delays (see Smulders et al., 1999).

In addition to latency differences, ERP research has shown two other types of important findings related to cognitive aging: (a) Older adults show permanence of responses to task-irrelevant stimuli that are typically suppressed in younger adults (e.g., Yamaguchi & Knight, 1991; Fabiani & Friedman, 1995; Fabiani et al., 2006); and (b) the scalp distribution of several ERP components, most notably the P300, appears to change with age (e.g., Yamaguchi & Knight, 1991; Fabiani & Friedman, 1995). The first finding is consistent with the presence of impairments in inhibitory processes and increased distractibility often reported in aging. The second finding is probably related to a change in the relative balance of different brain structures contributing to the scalp ERPs that are observed in aging.

Neuroimaging Evidence

The scalp distribution changes and the reduced suppression of some ERP responses to repeated or to-be-ignored stimuli resonate with the most commonly reported findings from the neuroimaging studies of cognitive aging (based on positron emission tomography [PET] and functional magnetic resonance imaging [fMRI]). This research has pointed out that aging is associated not only with a decrement of activity in some brain areas, but also with an increase in others. The earliest results of this type focused on the presence of bilateral responses in older adults in conditions

3

typically eliciting unilateral responses in younger adults (Cabeza et al., 1997; Reuter-Lorenz et al., 2000). Subsequent findings have shown that this phenomenon is more general—and may be caused by a balance shift between brain structures more directly related to signal processing and structures more related to elaborative processing (see Cabeza, 2002 for a review). Some investigators (e.g., Cabeza, 2002) have proposed that these changes in brain activity are strategic and that they reflect compensatory efforts employed by older adults to remediate for some deficit in cognitive abilities.

The interpretation of these effects is still largely debated. In the remainder of this chapter we focus on some of our own work in the area of functional brain changes associated with cognitive aging—work that in large part stresses the mechanisms that may underlie these changes rather than their hypothesized purposes. As our work has been based on combining several different measures of brain function, we first briefly review these different measures and emphasize their advantages and limitations.

Brain Imaging Methods
for the Study of Cognitive Aging

In considering how brain imaging methods can be useful to assess models of cognitive aging, we base our analysis on a general framework assuming that stimuli and tasks requirements induce activity in the brain that, in a general sense, flows from sensory to association to motor areas. This flow involves the orderly activation of some areas and inhibition of others, and, especially during familiar or sustained tasks, may be influenced by top-down control processes emphasizing certain types of cognitive activities over others. We assume that in aging, for various and to some extent not completely specified reasons, this normal flow may be sometimes disrupted, perhaps because of increased delays and variability in the completion of processes, reduced excitatory and/or inhibitory influences over particular areas. These changes may in turn induce the recruitment, either automatic or voluntary (as mediated by strategic choices), of processing routes that may be different from those used by younger adults. All of the theories already discussed can be encompassed by this framework. Thus, it would appear particularly useful that our measurement approach can provide this type of description at multiple levels within the system.

This description of the information flow would clearly benefit from brain imaging methods that combine good spatial and temporal resolution. These methods would allow us to localize functional slowing and detect changes in the processing flow, thus affording direct visualization of the phenomena predicted by different theories.

Currently, three main groups of noninvasive techniques are used to monitor brain activity during the performance of cognitive tasks. The first group includes electrophysiological methods, such as ERPs and magneto-encephalography (MEG). These methods image the electrical activity of large populations of neurons that are activated synchronously, and therefore possess a very good (millisecond level) temporal resolution. However, they are limited in their spatial resolution (several centimeters) because the electrical signal is smeared by the conductive properties of the head tissues, and different sources that overlap in time and space become difficult to separate. A second group of techniques includes hemodynamic imaging methods, such as fMRI, O^{15}-PET, and optical methods based on slow hemodynamic signals (near-infrared spectroscopy, NIRS; Villringer & Chance, 1997). These methods provide good spatial resolution (from a few centimeters to a few millimeters, depending on the method), but are limited in their temporal resolution (typically to a few seconds, or at best several hundred milliseconds) because they are based on the intrinsically slow hemodynamic signal associated with vasodilation occurring in active brain areas. A third group of techniques, introduced only recently, includes fast optical imaging methods (e.g., the event-related optical signal, or EROS; Gratton et al., 1995; Gratton & Fabiani, 2001). These methods measure changes in the optical properties of brain tissue that occur synchronously with neuronal activity. They provide very good temporal resolution (millisecond level) with subcentimeter spatial resolution (Gratton & Fabiani, 2003). For this reason, EROS appears to be a particularly promising technique for studying cognitive aging. Its major limitations include reduced penetration—so that structures located deep inside the brain cannot be imaged—and relatively poor signal-to-noise ratio (especially compared to hemodynamic methods).

It is important to consider that age-related brain changes may be at least in part linked to other physiological changes that often occur with aging—especially those affecting the vascular system and cardiopulmonary function. The importance of these factors is obvious in the case of stroke and other major cardiovascular disorders, including vascular dementia. However, even in nonpathological conditions these factors may play a significant role, as shown by both animal and human research reviewed in chapter 5 of this book. When hemodynamic brain imaging tools are used, these physiological changes may be particularly important, as changes in the observed brain activity could potentially be due to (a) actual changes in brain function, (b) changes in the observed signal that are not reflected in functional brain changes, or (c) changes in both of these phenomena—so that the relationship between neuronal and hemodynamic effects is changed compared to that in younger adults. In other words, changes in hemodynamic responses may be observed in older adults compared to younger adults, or in older adults differing in terms of their cardiovascular and cardiopulmonary function. In evaluating this research it is important to determine the extent to which these changes are related to neuronal function or limited to the hemodynamic responses associated with neuronal activity. This means that it is important to study how the relationship between neuronal and hemodynamic activity (the *neurovascular coupling;* Villringer & Dirnagl, 1995) changes with age.

Individual Differences as a Tool for Studying Aging

A number of ERP studies have highlighted the fact that some brain responses to repeated or to-be-ignored stimuli are not suppressed in older adults, whereas they are in younger adults. These findings are in line with a view of cognitive aging emphasizing reduced inhibitory processes and attention control, with subsequent increased distractibility. These effects, in turn, may stem from diminished top-down inhibitory feedback from attention control areas—such as dorsolateral prefrontal cortex. These areas are known to be particularly affected by aging in terms of tissue shrinkage (see West, 1996 for a review), which may explain reduced function. In the following sections, we briefly review some of these findings.

Early Sensory Brain Responses

One of the most commonly reported phenomena in cognitive aging is increased distractibility (Rabbitt, 1965). The task performance of older adults may be impaired by the presence of irrelevant distracters. This behavioral phenomenon has a clear physiological counterpart exemplified by the brain activity elicited by irrelevant auditory stimuli. When presented with repeated irrelevant stimulation, young adults quickly suppress their cortical responses to these stimuli (Sable et al., 2004). This process appears to a large extent to be the result of active suppression (requiring approximately 400 ms to occur), and is weakened in subjects with frontal lobe lesions (Knight et al., 1980; Knight & Grabowecky, 1995).

Recent studies (Alain & Woods, 1999; Fabiani et al., 2006; Golob et al., 2001) suggest that this suppression process may be impaired in older adults. For instance, Fabiani and colleagues (2006) presented short trains of five irrelevant auditory stimuli to young and old (age >65 years) adults while they were reading a book of their choice and after they had been told to ignore the sounds. Young adults showed a rapid suppression of the brain response elicited by the auditory stimuli in the train, demonstrated by a sharp reduction of the N1 component of the auditory evoked potential starting with the second stimulus in each train and continuing through the fifth and last stimulus. In contrast, old adults showed only a small reduction after the first stimulus and kept producing large N1 responses to all the stimuli in each train. This result suggests an inability to suppress irrelevant information, consistent with the reduced-inhibition account of cognitive aging proposed by Hasher and Zacks (1988). In turn, this could lead to interference with the normal processing of relevant information. Indeed, very recently we obtained preliminary data showing some evidence of this interference, as indicated by a correlation between the extent to which the N1 response is suppressed and older adults' performance in a concurrent primary task (Kazmerski et al., 2005), highlighting the role of individual differences in attention control. In our study (Fabiani et al., 2006) we also recorded fast optical imaging data. These data indicated the occurrence of activity in secondary auditory cortex (BA 41) whose suppression characteristics were very similar to those of the N1 ERP response.

Preattentive Processing of Changes in Stimulus Features

The data summarized in the previous section suggest that cognitive aging may be related to difficulties in attention-filtering mechanisms. A question that may arise is whether brain measures associated with preattentive processes would then also be influenced by aging. An ERP component associated with these types of processes that has been studied extensively is the mismatch negativity (MMN; Ritter et al., 1995). The MMN is a brain response to auditory stimuli that deviate in some way from an expected pattern, and it is obtained by subtracting the response to repeated (standard) sounds from those of rarely occurring (deviant) sounds. These stimuli need not be attended to; and in fact in most studies of the MMN, participants are instructed to ignore the stimuli and perform an unrelated task. For this reason the view is that the MMN taps into preattentive mismatch-detection processes and provides an index of sensory memory.

Conflicting reports exist in the literature about whether aging leads to a change in the MMN: Some authors report a reduction in amplitude (Czigler et al., 1992; Gaeta et al., 1998; Kazmerski et al., 1997; Woods, 1992) whereas others do not report significant differences with age, at least at short interstimulus intervals (Pekkonen et al., 1996). Part of the variation may stem from the fact that the hearing threshold for older adults may be markedly higher than that of young adults. To eliminate this confound, we ran an MMN study in which the auditory threshold was measured on each individual subject before ERPs were recorded, and stimuli were adjusted in intensity to reflect changes in auditory thresholds (Sable et al., in preparation). The results indicated that the response to the deviant stimuli obtained in young and old adults in this case is virtually identical. This suggests that the processing of deviant information per se is not influenced significantly by age. However, similarly to what is shown by the N1 data summarized previously, it appears that the processing of the repeated standards is not fully suppressed in older adults, thus resulting in a smaller MMN when the standard waveforms are subtracted from the deviant waveforms.

Age-Related Changes in the P300 Response

The P300 is a large ERP component typically most positive at parietal and central locations and with a peak latency exceeding 300 ms (Fabiani et al., 2007). Since its discovery (Sutton et al., 1965), the P300 has been linked to attentional and control processes, as well as to allocation of working memory resources. In particular, research by Donchin and colleagues (e.g., Squires et al., 1977) demonstrated that the amplitude of P300 is very sensitive to the subjective probability of a particular stimulus, which in turn is influenced by the local stimulus sequence. For instance, in a random series of two possible stimuli, P300 is larger if the eliciting stimulus differs from the preceding stimuli (e.g., the last stimulus of the sequence BBBA produces a larger P300 than the last stimulus of the sequence AAAA). In fact, an apparent exception to this rule occurs when a series of alternations occurs (ABABA vs. ABABB): In this case the P300 is larger when the alternation is violated (Squires et al., 1977). These findings led Donchin (1981; see also Donchin & Coles, 1988) to propose that in these types of tasks, (a) subjects maintain a representation of the current stimulus sequence; (b) P300 is related to the processes that are required when the current stimulus violates the expectancies based on the sequence; (c) these processes reflect a refreshing of stimulus representations that may have decayed over time or as a function of interference ("context updating hypothesis"). These updating processes are more needed in cases in which the representations have decayed than when the representations are still active—and they are reflected in variations in the amplitude of P300. It can be hypothesized that subjects with higher working memory capacity (or better resistance to interference) should need these updating processes less than subjects with lower working memory capacity. An initial finding of this type was reported by Klein and colleagues (1984) in subjects with perfect pitch (who did not produce a P300 when presented with rare auditory stimuli).

In our case, we were interested in determining whether individual differences in working memory capacity in young and old adults could also predict differences in P300 amplitude as a function of stimulus sequence. Specifically, we (Brumback et al., 2005a) predicted that subjects with high Operation-span scores (O-span is a test developed by Randy Engle and colleagues [Kane & Engle, 2000] to evaluate working memory capacity in the presence of interference) should produce a smaller P300 in the case of stimulus sequence violations than subjects with low O-span scores. The results supported this prediction. While this original study was conducted in young adults, we have now replicated the same finding in older subjects (Brumback et al., 2005b). This suggests that the factors underlying individual differences in working memory processes in young and old adults are similar and may exert their effects throughout the life span.

Other parameters of P300 have been investigated extensively in aging. One is P300 latency, which typically shows an increase of 1 or 2 ms per year of age starting from young adulthood (Polich et al., 1985). Whereas this finding is very robust and consistent with a processing-slowing view of cognitive aging, it should be noted that large individual differences occur, so that the variability in P300 latency in old adults is greater than in young adults. The factors underlying this variability have not been investigated in detail yet.

It is not only the amplitude and latency of P300 that vary with age, but also its distribution over the scalp (e.g., Fabiani & Friedman, 1995); young adults exhibit a P300 with a clear parictal focus, whereas old adults have a larger positivity over frontal scalp locations relative to their parietal P300 response. This finding is intriguing because the scalp distribution of an ERP component is typically considered to be dependent on the brain areas responsible for its generation. A change in scalp distribution is taken to indicate that different configurations of brain areas are responsible for the P300 observed at the scalp in young and old adults. In their work, Fabiani and Friedman (1995) showed that young adults also exhibit a frontal distribution for P300 during the first few trials of a study. However, this frontal activity (which is likely to indicate orienting responses to novel stimuli; Knight, 1984) subsides rapidly over the course of the experiment in young adults, whereas it persists in the old adults. This finding is reminiscent of the N1 effects described earlier: Old adults show persistence of responses that are quickly suppressed in young adults. This early frontal activity in fact resembles another ERP component, the P3a or Novelty P3 (e.g., Knight, 1984), which is elicited by unique, novel, and never-repeated items. In a subsequent paper, Fabiani and colleagues (1998) reported that not all old adults show this phenomenon to the same extent. Those showing a "younger-looking" P300 also performed better on several neuropsychological tasks, such as the Wisconsin Card Sorting Task (WCST). It is likely that these differences reflect lack of flexibility and inability to suppress inappropriate responses and brain processes.

In summary, the P300 data indicate clear differences not only between young and old adults, but also within old adults. These differences appear to reflect variations in processing speed (P300 latency effects), working memory capacity (sequential effects on P300 amplitude), and lack of inhibition (scalp distribution effects).

Research on Brain Connectivity

The brain is a complex network, and within it cognitive processes can be expected to reflect the coordinated action of a variety of cortical areas. This coordination may be affected by aging because of mistiming of the activities of different areas (related to slowing phenomena), lack of appropriate inhibitory processes, and impaired connectivity between different areas. Connectivity can be considered at two levels: (a) anatomical and (b) functional or effective. Anatomical connectivity refers to the fiber tracts connecting different brain and cortical regions. These tracts may be affected by the aging process because of diminished functionality of the originating cells or decreased myelination or both. Effective connectivity refers to the relative effect that activity in one area has on another area. However, because causality is often difficult to infer, most investigators refer to functional rather than effective connectivity, which can be expressed as the correlation in activity between cortical areas. Since processing may be expected to flow across different brain regions over time, it is possible that correlations between areas may be manifested with some lag.

The last few years have seen a large growth in studies of structural and functional brain connectivity (for a review see Rykhlevskaia et al., 2008). We have recently begun exploring the effects of age on these phenomena, exploiting the combined spatial and temporal resolution of EROS, which allows us to provide independent estimates of the time course of activity in regions of the brain that are as close to each other as 2 cm. In this work (Gratton et al., in press; Rykhlevskaia et al., 2006) we used a paradigm in which subjects were asked to categorize a stimulus according to either its spatial or its verbal properties. The relevant dimension for a particular trial was identified by a cue presented shortly (2 s) before this stimulus. Our focus was on the preparatory brain activity following the cue. Specifically, we were interested in those conditions in which the cue signaled the subjects that the relevant dimension was changed with respect to the previous trial *(switch trials)*. We compared this condition to that in which the cue did not signal a dimension change *(no-switch trials)*. As older adults typically show less flexibility than young adults, we expected the switch trials to produce longer reaction times (as was the case). Further, we expected the switch cue to elicit activity in prefrontal areas, related to the activation of appropriate classification rules and inhibition of inappropriate ones. Because we were contrasting spatial and verbal classification rules, we expected right-hemisphere activation in the case of switch-to-spatial rules, and left-hemisphere activation in the case of switch-to-verbal rules. This was in fact the pattern of results we obtained in young subjects; older adults, however, showed a bilateral pattern, consistent with the many recent imaging studies indicating bilateral brain activity in old adults in cases in which unilateral brain activity is observed in young adults.

Most interestingly, however, we also observed a relationship between these phenomena and brain anatomy. Specifically, we observed that the switch cost in reaction time was correlated with the size of the anterior third of the corpus callosum (measured from structural magnetic resonance images), the most important fiber tract connecting the two hemispheres in the brain: Subjects with a larger corpus callosum showed smaller switch costs than subjects with a small corpus callosum. The corpus callosum was reduced in size in the older adults, but the effect of corpus callosum size on behavior was larger than the effect of age per se. The size of the corpus callosum also had an effect on the correlation between left- and right-hemisphere functional activity (measured with EROS): Subjects with a large corpus callosum showed a younger-looking pattern as well as large negative lagged correlations between the two hemispheres (possibly indicating inhibition of the "incorrect" rules), and these negative correlations were reduced in subjects with a small corpus callosum. These data suggest that corpus callosum size may be a very good predictor of difficulties in task-switching when the task is likely to activate alternate homologous areas across the two hemispheres (such as those supporting preparation for verbal and spatial rules). Further, they suggest that the effect of age on task-switching may be at least in part mediated by its effect on the size of corpus callosum (and perhaps other white matter tracts). Finally, the data also suggest that one of the effects of the reduction in corpus callosum may be a reduction of interhemispheric inhibitory processes. An interesting question is whether this is only a particular case of a general reduction in inhibitory connections between brain regions with aging, consistent with the reduced-inhibition hypothesis (Hasher & Zacks, 1988).

Research on Neurovascular Coupling

As mentioned earlier, the study of neurovascular coupling may be particularly important in the study of aging. There are two reasons for this: (a) Age-related changes in neurovascular coupling (if substantiated) may influence hemodynamic measures of brain function, such as fMRI, PET, and NIRS; and (b) potentially, changes in neurovascular coupling may render the aging brain less able to cope with high processing demands, especially if they are sustained over time.

Recently we have begun exploiting the capability of optical methods to image concurrently neuronal (scattering) and hemodynamic (absorption) signals. We have conducted two studies in this area. The first was a pilot project conducted on eight young adults (Gratton et al., 2001). The use of a monochromatic recording system (750 nm) did not allow a spectroscopic approach, and therefore the slow hemodynamic effects could not be decomposed into oxy- and deoxy-hemoglobin effects. The experiment, based on visual stimulation, involved several stimulation frequencies (see

11

Fox & Raichle, 1985 for a similar approach for PET measures). The main result of this study was that the slow hemodynamic effect was proportional to the size of the fast scattering effect integrated over time in young adults. The study further indicated that fast and slow signals colocalized to the same brain volume.

The second study (Fabiani et al., 2005) was a larger-scale experiment based on the same paradigm, conducted on 64 young and old adults differing in cardiopulmonary fitness. The study used a spectroscopic approach based on multiple light wavelengths, and used both fMRI and visual evoked potentials recordings as external validation criteria. Preliminary results from this study replicated and extended those of the first study. As in the first study, a relatively linear relationship was observed between the fast EROS response and slow effect (measured in terms of oxy-hemoglobin concentration changes). All three groups of subjects showed a relatively similar fast EROS response. However, the slope of the neurovascular function was reduced (by approximately 50%) in old adults in the low cardiopulmonary fitness group. This finding was due to a marked reduction of the oxy-hemoglobin response in this group.

The results of this second study emphasize that neurovascular coupling may change with age, in particular as a function of cardiopulmonary fitness. This finding suggests that down regulation of hemodynamic responses in aging may not necessarily imply a reduction in neuronal responses. However, it is important to note that other results obtained with imaging methods in older subjects, such as recruitment of additional cortical regions (Cabeza, 2002), cannot be accounted for solely by a reduction in neurovascular coupling.

Summary and Future Directions

The data reviewed here show substantial psychophysiological and brain imaging evidence for the three postulated accounts of cognitive aging (slowing of processing, reduced inhibition, and reduction in working memory). Using a connectivity framework, these three mechanisms can be seen as largely overlapping: Both processing slowing and reduced inhibition can be viewed as the outcome of connectivity problems in aging, and the deficit in working memory can be viewed as determined by interference effects caused by lack of suppression of irrelevant information. Thus, the psychophysiological data provide a unifying view of the effects of cognitive aging.

Another important feature of the studies reviewed here is the role of individual differences. Most of the phenomena observed in aging vary greatly between individuals; some subjects maintain a performance level and a profile of psychophysiological and brain imaging data very similar to those of young adults, and others show marked differences. These individual differences appear to rely in part on anatomical (e.g., corpus callosum size) and cardiopulmonary differences between individuals (as shown in our work on neurovascular coupling). Indeed, recent data from our lab (Gordon et al., 2008) and other labs (Colcombe et al., 2005) indicate that the anatomical changes may also be mediated by cardiopulmonary fitness level. In our work, we also show profound individual differences in working memory span and neuropsychological variables, all correlated to ERP and brain imaging results. The extent to which these individual differences can be accounted for by cardiopulmonary fitness level remains to be determined and will be the subject of future research. It is also likely that other factors, such as education, other aspects of lifestyle, and the genome may play significant roles in determining variations in the cognitive aging process. However, the study of anatomical and functional changes in the flow of information through the brain promises to generate useful descriptions of this critical phenomenon.

CHAPTER 2

The Effects of the Cognitive Complexity of Occupational Conditions and Leisure-Time Activities on the Intellectual Functioning of Older Adults

Carmi Schooler, PhD

*Section on Socioenvironmental Studies, Intramural Research Program,
National Institute of Mental Health, National Institutes of Health,
Department of Health and Human Services*

In this review I focus on the effects of complexity of paid work and leisure-time activities on older people's intellectual functioning. In doing so I hope to provide evidence that even late in the life course, carrying out intellectually demanding tasks both on and off of the job positively affects intellectual functioning. Establishing the existence of such a cognitive effect of occupational and nonoccupational conditions should be of direct interest to those concerned with understanding how the environment affects the psychological functioning of older people. At a practical level, establishing such a relationship could provide useful insights into designing programs and environments that would improve the life experience of the elderly.

Plausible, yet contradictory, hypotheses exist about the effects of intellectually demanding activities on the cognitive functioning of normal older adults. On the one hand, there are reasons to believe that older individuals would be more adversely affected than younger ones by intellectually demanding environmental conditions. If cognitive speed (Salthouse, 1991) or working memory (Baddeley, 1986), or both, decline with age, one might predict that older workers would react poorly to such demanding environmental conditions. On the other hand, the very existence of such deficits might make it more important for older than for younger individuals to be in environments in which they must continue to practice and develop their intellectual skills.

As we shall see, a fair amount of evidence demonstrates the existence of a correlation between elderly individuals' levels of intellectual functioning and the intellectual demand of the tasks they perform. The core problem is discerning the direction of causal effects that underlie this correlation.

Any given correlation between relatively high levels of cognitive function and participation in a particular cognitively demanding activity can be, on the one hand, the result of dealing with the cognitive demands imposed by that activity. On the other hand, such a correlation may be the result of having characteristics that increase the likelihood of choosing, or having been chosen, to engage and stay engaged in that activity. At its most basic level, the question is the extent to which such a correlation results from the effect of the characteristics of the environment on the characteristics of the person and how much of the correlation results from the plausible reciprocal effect of the characteristics of the person on the environment.

There are really only two basic ways of dealing with this issue: (1) experimentation and (2) complex statistical modeling of longitudinal data, for example structural equation modeling (SEM)—neither of which is perfect. Experiments, in which subjects are randomly assigned to relevant experimental conditions, are almost invariably limited in (a) the types and numbers of participants that can be used and (b) the power, length, and appropriateness of the manipulations. Statistical modeling, in turn, is limited by (a) an inability to completely rule out the possibility that some variable not included in the model is at work either in terms of selecting individuals into particular environments or because a given set of environmental conditions may have different effects on different types of individuals, and (b) the intractability of certain types and distributions of data to appropriate statistical manipulation. Given the limitations of both types of approach, it is my belief that, at present, the best estimates of the effects of environmental conditions on the intellectual functioning of elderly individuals in the real world is provided by statistical modeling of longitudinal data.

The earliest SEM-based findings on the effects of environmental conditions on intellectual functioning come from the Kohn-Schooler (1983) research program on the psychological effects of occupational conditions carried out on a representative sample of U.S. workers first interviewed in 1964 and then reinterviewed in 1974. In this chapter, I will (1) describe the early Kohn-Schooler U.S. studies and tests of the generalizability of their findings in other industrial societies; (2) discuss other relatively recent relevant studies that do not directly face the issue of plausible reciprocal effects, including studies on both normal individuals and those showing clinically significant cognitive decline; (3) detail more recent studies based on a 1994 reinterview of the 1974 Kohn-Schooler sample that extend the earlier findings outside of the workplace as well as 20 years further along the life course; and (4) discuss some human quasi-experimental studies that lend further support to the findings and provide some insight into relevant cognitive and neuropsychobiological mechanisms.

Earlier Kohn-Schooler Studies of Environmental Complexity and Intellectual Functioning

The early Kohn-Schooler research program (Kohn & Schooler, 1978, 1983) explored the potential reciprocal or cross-lagged effects (or both) of occupational conditions and psychological functioning. In terms of cognitive functioning, its central hypothesis was that doing cognitively complex self-directed work has a positive effect on intellectual functioning, and doing cognitively simple non-self-directed work has a negative effect. The researchers also hypothesized that individuals' levels of intellectual functioning reciprocally affected the cognitive demand level of their environments because individuals would be relatively more likely to choose to, be chosen to, and continue to participate in activities whose cognitive demands matched their intellectual capacities. In most of these studies, the use of SEM permitted the estimation of nonrecursive reciprocal-effects models that tested the degree to which the correlation between an environmental condition and a psychological characteristic reflected the effect of the environmental condition on that psychological characteristic—as compared to the degree to which having that characteristic leads to choosing or keeping that environmental condition.

Job Complexity and Intellectual Functioning

The most extensively studied environmental complexity factor in the Kohn-Schooler research program was the substantive complexity of paid work. In terms of its effect on intellectual functioning, the program's central longitudinal finding was that job conditions offering challenge and opportunity for doing self-directed substantively complex work increase men's intellectual flexibility: Work conditions that limit intellectual challenge and self-direction on the job decrease men's intellectual flexibility (Kohn & Schooler, 1983). Kohn and Schooler also found a significant lagged effect of earlier intellectual functioning on the subsequent substantive complexity of men's paid work, suggesting a reciprocal relationship over time between complexity of work done and psychological functioning.

Several other nonlongitudinal studies from the Kohn-Schooler research program and its overseas extensions provided further support for the hypothesized causal connection between complex, cognitively demanding work conditions and intellectual functioning. These included studies of U.S. women's paid work (Miller, Schooler, Kohn, & Miller, 1979; Kohn & Schooler, 1983, chapter 8), as well as studies of paid work in Japan (Naoi & Schooler, 1985, 1990; Schooler & Naoi, 1988), Poland (Kohn &

Slomczynski, 1990), and Ukraine (Kohn et al., 1997). The same relationship between substantively complex work and intellectual flexibility was also found in other types of work, such as school work (Miller, Kohn, & Schooler, 1986) and women's housework (Schooler, Miller, Miller, & Richtand, 1984; Kohn & Schooler, 1983, chapter 10).

A particularly relevant finding comes from Miller, Slomczynski, and Kohn's (1985) analyses of the causal connection between substantively complex work and intellectual flexibility in different age cohorts in both the United States and Poland. Using SEM to estimate reciprocal-effects models with the data from the Kohn-Schooler U.S. survey and its Polish replication, Miller, Slomczynski, and Kohn found that in both countries, substantively complex work increases intellectual flexibility in both younger and older cohorts. Taking into account the overall pattern of their findings, particularly with their U.S. sample (i.e., the 1964-1974 Kohn-Schooler sample), Miller, Slomczynski, and Kohn suggest that "the reciprocal effects of the substantive complexity and ideational flexibility are not only as strong for older as for younger men, but may even be stronger for older men" (p. 609). What clearly differed among the cohorts was the substantive complexity of the work done. In both countries, older workers did less substantively complex work.

The Kohn-Schooler research program also provided evidence that the intellectual demand level of occupational conditions can affect the intellectual demand level of off-the-job experiences. Using data from the Kohn-Schooler study, Miller and Kohn (1983) compared the degree to which doing substantively complex work on the job increases the intellectual complexity of leisure-time activities with the degree to which having intellectually complex leisure-time activities increases the substantive complexity of work done on the job. They found both reciprocal causal paths to be significant. As expected, given the greater control that individuals would seem to have over the nature of their leisure-time activities than of their jobs, the path from the substantive complexity of individuals' leisure-time activities to the substantive complexity of their work was significantly smaller than its reciprocal. These conclusions hold true even when individuals' levels of intellectual functioning are controlled.

Leisure Activities and Intellectual Functioning

Although the studies just outlined did not directly link leisure-time activity to intellectual functioning, a recent study that has its historical origins in the Kohn-Schooler research program provides evidence suggesting that the complexity of leisure activities has a positive effect on intellectual functioning. On the basis of research carried out in Eastern Europe, Kohn and colleagues (2000) found that the complexity of activities outside, as well as within, paid employment is linked to intellectual flexibility. Kohn and colleagues found that this empirical connection existed even under the conditions of radical social change typifying Poland as it moved from a socialist to a capitalist economy in the winter of 1992. They uncovered very specific empirical links, not only between intellectual flexibility and the substantive complexity of men's and women's paid employment and women's housework, but also between intellectual flexibility and the complexity of both male and female pensioners' activities. The absence of longitudinal data in their East European study deterred Kohn and colleagues from using SEM to estimate reciprocal-effects SEM models that would assess the causal patterns underlying these relationships. In the absence of such analyses, they make the case that the consonance of their findings with those of longitudinal and simulated longitudinal analyses of past studies strongly suggests that these relationships, too, are reciprocal.

In sum, the Kohn-Schooler research program provides clear evidence for the existence of reciprocal effects between the substantive complexity of paid work and intellectual functioning of individuals in various societies. Related cross-cultural studies have also provided evidence that substantive complexity of work and leisure-time activities is clearly related to better intellectual functioning. More generally, even two decades ago, the results from the earlier Kohn-Schooler occupational studies were consistent with a large body of research then available from a wide range of disciplines, including cognitive aging and animal-based neurobiology studies, which strongly suggested that exposure to complex environments increases intellectual functioning throughout the life course and across species (Schooler, 1984). In the following section, I review relatively recent studies from other research groups aimed at investigating the relationship between environmental complexity and cognitive functioning in older people.

Other Studies Linking Environmental Complexity and Intellectual Functioning

Interest in the effects of environmental factors on aging has sparked a great deal of research directed at the correlates or determinants of cognitive functioning among older people with or without dementia or other degenerative diseases. Although the findings from these studies are not completely consistent, the preponderance of the evidence is quite consistent with the hypothesis that exposure to enriched or intellectually challenging environments has a positive effect on intellectual functioning among older people. There is, however, a caveat that hinders our fully accepting these findings as proof of this hypothesis. Although sometimes longitudinal, these studies tend to employ research approaches that focus on testing for the existence of relationships between environmental conditions and cognitive functioning while controlling for the effects of other potentially relevant factors (e.g., education). The research approaches they employ, however, do not directly explore the potential reciprocal relationships between environmental complexity and intellectual functioning. Consequently, these studies do not rule out the possibility that the relationships observed are due to the greater likelihood that relatively intelligent individuals will be selected into, and selectively stay in, relatively intellectually demanding environments.

Environmental Complexity and Normal Cognitive Functioning

Various studies have examined the relationship across the lifespan between individuals' cognitive functioning and the cognitive demands of their occupations. Others have similarly looked at the relationship between individuals' cognitive functioning and the demands of their leisure-time activities. Although not logically conclusive, the evidence is congruent with the hypothesis that carrying cognitively demanding leisure-time activities either on the job or in leisure time has a positive effect on intellectual funtioning—while non-cognitively demanding environmental demands have the opposite effect.

Job Complexity and Normal Cognitive Functioning

Using nonlongitudinal data collected by the U.S. Employment Service, Avolio and Waldman examined the relationship between the cognitive demand level of jobs and intellectual functioning across the life span. In their first paper, they showed a significant positive correlation between the intellectual functioning of workers and job complexity (Avolio & Waldman, 1990). In their second paper (Avolio & Waldman, 1994), they showed a positive relationship between workers' intellectual functioning and a fairly rough measure of the cognitive demands of their occupations, even when age, race, and gender, and education were taken into account. In neither paper was there a significant interaction among age, job cognitive demand level, and intellectual functioning. The absence of such an interaction suggests that the relationships between cognitive functioning and the cognitive demands of job conditions as indexed by Avolio and Waldman do not vary with age. More generally, according to Avolio and Waldman's conclusion, their findings suggest that there "may be unique factors in the work context that affect the maintenance of abilities, the decline of abilities or both across the life span" (p. 438, 1994).

In a prospective study, Bosma and colleagues (2003) explored the relationships between mental workload, educational attainment, and cognitive functioning among 708 Dutch men and women aged 50 to 80. The authors coded the self-reported description of the study participants' current or most recent job using a scheme similar to that of the U.S. *Dictionary of Occupational Titles*. A mental workload score was then assigned to each job category depending on responses to questions about whether or not the job was mentally demanding and required strong concentration, great precision, and working under time pressure. The study revealed two important findings: (1) Lower levels of educational attainment and cognitive workload at baseline were significantly associated with stronger decline in longitudinal cognitive functioning, measured by differences in scores on processing speed, memory, and a general cognitive status examination; and (2) cognitive workload accounted for 42% of the effect of educational attainment on cognitive functioning. The authors concluded that providing work-related cognitive stimuli and challenges for poorly educated people might help in reducing the age-related gap in cognitive decline between poorly and highly educated people.

Leisure Activities and Normal Cognitive Functioning

Bosma and colleagues (2002) provided some evidence for the potential reciprocal effects between leisure-time activities and cognitive functioning among 830 nondemented middle- and old-aged men and women in The Netherlands. In this three-year longitudinal study, the authors estimated two separate regression models. In the first model, level of leisure activities at baseline was related to follow-up cognitive functioning, even when age, sex, educational level, and baseline cognitive functioning were controlled. In the second model, cognitive functioning at baseline was related to follow-up leisure activities, with baseline age, sex, educational level, and leisure activities controlled for. Bosma and colleagues found a positive relationship between leisure activities and cognitive functioning. They consequently suggested that stimulating individuals to participate in leisure activities may prevent the development of adverse cognitive functioning that in turn would affect participation in leisure activities. Although the authors did not test the reciprocal effects in the same model simultaneously, their findings are congruent with the hypothesis (Schooler, 1984, 1990) that environmental complexity has a positive effect on intellectual functioning throughout the life span.

In two other papers based on longitudinal data sets unrelated to the Kohn-Schooler studies, the authors report having tested the Schooler environmental complexity hypothesis with apparently conflicting results: supported versus not supported. Pushkar Gold and colleagues (1995) see their analyses of data from the Canadian Army Veterans Study as supporting the hypothesis by demonstrating that an engaged lifestyle, which they specifically link to exposure to complex environments, has a positive effect on intellectual functioning late in life. Hultsch, Hertzog, Small, and Dixon (1999), using data from the Victoria Longitudinal Study, view their analyses as not providing strong support for the environmental complexity hypothesis. They reach this conclusion because a model in which exposure to environmental complexity increases intellectual functioning fits their data no better than a model proposing the reverse, that high levels of intellectual functioning increase exposure to complex environments. In addition, Hultsch and colleagues (1999) reexamine the Canadian Veterans data of Pushkar Gold and colleagues (1995) and conclude that when properly analyzed, this data set also supports their conclusion that the effect of level of intellectual functioning on participation in complex lifestyle activities is stronger than the reverse effect reported by Pushkar and colleagues (1995). These conclusions led to a round of conflicting comments by the two sets of authors (Hertzog, Hultsch, & Dixon, 1999; Pushkar et al., 1999), with each side staunchly defending its position. Although the findings of both studies are congruent with the existence of a reciprocal causal connection between exposure to complex environments and relatively high level intellectual functioning, neither study directly evaluated this possibility.

In a recent cross-sectional study exploring the relationship between cognitive stimulation and cognitive functioning among adults aged 20 to 80, Salthouse, Berish, and Miles (2002) claim to have found no evidence that engaging in cognitively stimulating activities and cognitive functioning are related and, therefore, no support for the hypothesis that cognitive stimulation preserves or enhances functioning that would otherwise decline with age. Their findings are in sharp contrast with the growing evidence that supports the positive effects of dealing with complex environments on cognitive functioning. By the authors' admission, the cross-sectional nature of the study and the fact that the study participants were relatively highly educated and healthy may have underestimated the relationships between cognitive stimulation and cognitive functioning. Of at least equal concern is that their measure of cognitive stimulation was a subjective one—based on the respondents' own judgment of the cognitive demand level of the activities in which they participated. It seems more than plausible that this subjectivity may have seriously affected the results, since there is every reason to believe that individuals' ratings of the cognitive demand of a given activity would be affected by their level of cognitive functioning.

In sum, with the exception of the work of Salthouse and colleagues (2002), the studies reviewed in this section provide support to, or are at least congruent with, the environmental complexity or the cognitive reserve hypothesis or both. Nevertheless, despite some efforts at estimating separate models to test each hypothesis, none of these studies deals forthrightly with the question of the degree to which correlations between levels of environmental complexity and intellectual functioning reflect the psychological effects of complex environments, or the degree to which individuals who function well intellectually select or are selected into such environments.

Environmental Complexity and Clinical Cognitive Decline

Paralleling the research on environmental complexity and normal cognitive functioning, a number of studies deal with environmental complexity and clinical cognitive decline. Some occupations and occupational conditions that may be linked to relatively less cognitive demand have been linked to various forms of clinical cognitive impairment in older peole. Similarly, participation in cognitively demanding leisure-time activities has been associated with reduced risk of such clinical conditions as Alzheimer's disease and senile dementia.

Job Complexity and Clinical Cognitive Decline

Indirect support for the hypothesis that carrying out intellectually demanding complex tasks on the job has a positive effect on intellectual functioning is provided by studies that link types of occupations with the incidence of clinically significant cognitive decline among older people. In a longitudinal Swedish study that followed 913 nondemented older people (aged 75 or more) for more than six years, Qiu and colleagues (2003) found the longest-held occupational position to be one of the predictors of the risk of Alzheimer's disease. Specifically, the authors found that having manual work as the longest-held occupational position, particularly work involving goods production, was associated with greater risk for Alzheimer's disease and all types of dementia than having nonmanual work. Although the authors speculated that exposure to a multitoxic work environment, poor socioeconomic conditions and lifestyle, and lower initial intelligence may be potential mechanisms underlying the association between manual work and the risk of Alzheimer's disease and dementia, other occupational mechanisms, such as the often-routine and cognitively less challenging nature of manual work, cannot be ruled out.

Several other studies from the United States and other industrialized societies have also shown a link between occupational conditions or categories and dementia among older populations. In the United States, Stern and colleagues (1994) followed 593 nondemented individuals 60 years or older for one to four years. They found that the risk of incidence of dementia was significantly higher among individuals with lower occupational attainment and education. They concluded that low levels of educational and occupational attainment factors may lower the individual's cognitive reserve—a reserve that might serve to delay the manifestation of dementia. In a longitudinal study in France, Dartigues and colleagues (1992) analyzed their baseline data from a large community sample (N = 3777) of people aged 65 and older. They found, after controlling for age, sex, educational level, and other covariates, that farm workers, domestic service employees, and blue-collar workers had a higher risk of cognitive impairment than did participants who had an "intellectual occupation." In a longitudinal analysis using the same sample, they found that female farmers had a higher risk of dementia compared to male and female professionals and managers (Helmer et al., 2001). No difference was found across occupations in the risk of Alzheimer's disease.

Although these studies provide evidence that links occupational conditions to cognitive functioning of older people, the researchers generally do not seem to have estimated the degree to which their findings reflect the relationship between cognitive level of performance and the likelihood of getting and keeping a job characterized by a given level of cognitive demand. Consequently, the direction of the causal connection underlying the observed correlations remains questionable. In addition, when the cognitive demand level of the work environment is estimated through the use of broad occupational categories, the level of occupational complexity is not directly measured, only assumed.

Leisure Activities and Clinical Cognitive Decline

Relevant studies also generally suggest a positive relationship between participation in leisure-time activities, particularly cognitively demanding ones, and nondemented cognitive functioning among older people. For instance, Wilson and colleagues (2002), using data from a sample of 801 Catholic nuns, priests, and brothers in the United States, tested the hypothesis that frequent participation in cognitive activities is associated with a reduced risk of Alzheimer's disease. The authors found that a unit of cognitive activity score at baseline, measured by seven common activities such as reading a newspaper, listening to radio, and reading books, was associated with a 33% reduction in risk of Alzheimer's disease approximately four years later at follow-up. In addition, with age, gender, education, and baseline cognitive functioning controlled for, a unit of increase in cognitive activity was associated with reduced general cognitive aging by 47%, reduced working memory by 60%, and reduced perceptual speed by 30%.

Similarly, Verghese and colleagues (2003) followed 469 older people in New York aged 75 years or above for about five years and examined the effects of leisure-time activities on the risk of dementia. The authors found participation in leisure activities to be associated with a reduced risk of dementia, even after controlling for baseline cognitive status, age, sex, educational level, and chronic medical illnesses. More importantly, the study revealed that it was participation in cognitively demanding leisure activities (e.g., reading, playing board games, and playing musical instruments), rather than participation in physical leisure activities, that had a positive effect on cognitive functioning.

Similar results have also been reported in studies from other industrial nations. Using data from 776 participants (aged 75 years and older) in a longitudinal population study in Stockholm, Wang and colleagues (2002) examined whether engagement in various leisure activities more than six years before the diagnosis of dementia was related to increased or decreased risk of the incidence of dementia. The authors found that frequent engagement in mental, social, or productive activities at baseline was inversely associated with the incidence of dementia. Not unlike the findings from the study by Verghese and colleagues (2003), the results of this study suggest that the participation of older people in socially and intellectually stimulating activities may be relevant in the preservation of their cognitive functioning. Another Swedish study has also shown that greater participation in overall leisure-time activities, including intellectual-cultural, self-empowering, and domestic activities, was associated with lower levels of risk for Alzheimer's disease and dementia 20 years later (Crowe et al., 2003). Interestingly, in this study greater participation in intellectual-cultural activities reduced the risk of Alzheimer's disease among female more than male participants.

Friedland and colleagues (2001) have also established that, compared to healthy case-controls, patients with Alzheimer's disease show reduced diversity of overall activities and intensity of intellectual activities at least five years prior to the onset of the disease. Healthy controls were found to be more active than Alzheimer's disease patients during their early adulthood (ages 20-39) as well as middle adulthood (ages 40-50) in all activity categories, including passive, social, and intellectual activities, even when age, gender, education, and income adequacy were taken into account. Nevertheless, the findings for middle adulthood hold true when early-adult leisure activity level is controlled for. The fact that spending relatively little leisure time in intellectually demanding activities in middle adulthood is predictive of Alzheimer's disease, even when the percentage of leisure time spent in such activities in early adulthood is controlled for, decreases the likelihood that the lower level of intellectual leisure-time activities in middle adulthood—characteristic of those who later develop Alzheimer's disease—is a function of some type of early-adulthood presymptomatic cognitive dysfunction such as that described in the Nun Study (Snowden et al., 1996).

All in all, the findings of the studies described here, which are generally representative of those in the literature, are strikingly congruent with the possibility that participating in relatively intellectually demanding leisure-time activities acts to decrease the likelihood of senile dementia, or delay the clinical signs of its occurrence, or both.

Recent Section on Socioenvironmental Studies' Research on Environmental Complexity and Intellectual Functioning

Several relatively recent projects from the National Institute of Mental Health Section on Socioenvironmental Studies (SSES) have specifically tested the possibility of reciprocal effects between environmental complexity and intellectual studies in older individuals (Schooler, Mulatu, & Oates, 1999; Schooler & Mulatu, 2001, Schooler, Mulatu, & Oates, 2004). These papers expanded the earlier Kohn-Schooler studies by examining the reciprocal relationships between the complexity of paid work (Schooler, Mulatu, and & Oates, 1999, 2004) or leisure-time activities (Schooler & Mulatu, 2001) and intellectual functioning using data collected in 1974 and in 1994-1995, when the original participants had aged by about 20 years. In order to provide the context to the discussion, the following sections briefly describe (1) the sample from which the longitudinal data for these studies were derived, (2) our measures of environmental complexity and intellectual functioning, (3) data analysis and major findings, and (4) significance of the findings.

Characteristics of the Longitudinal Sample

The first-wave data collection for the Kohn-Schooler study of the psychological effects of occupational conditions began in 1964, when a nationally representative sample (N = 3101) of employed men was interviewed. The sample was an area probability sample drawn by the National Opinion Research Center (NORC) of males over 16 years of age then currently employed at least 25 hr per week in nonmilitary occupations. In 1974, NORC interviewed a representative subsample of approximately one-fourth of the first-wave respondents who were less than 65 years old at that time. Of the 883 men who were randomly selected for the follow-up study, 820 (93%) were located. Of the 785 men who were still alive, 687 (88%) were interviewed. In addition, in the 1974 study, the wife of every male respondent who was then married was interviewed. Interviews were conducted with 555 women, 90% of the 617 eligible. They ranged in age from 26 to 65 years. In the 1994-1995 follow-up, we succeeded in locating 95% (650) of the 687 households that took part in the 1974 survey. Of the 1242 men and women interviewed in 1974, 707 (352 men and 355 women) were reinterviewed in 1994-1995; others were not located, had died, or did not complete the interview because of illness or refusal.

In our study examining the reciprocal effects of substantive complexity of paid work and intellectual functioning (Schooler, Mulatu, & Oates, 1999), we focused only on those people who worked both in 1974 and in 1994-1995. The effective sample size for this study was 233; 160 were males and 73 were females. The age range was 41 to 83 and the median age was 57; median level of education was high school graduate with some technical schooling.

In our analysis examining the reciprocal effects of cognitively demanding leisure-time activities and intellectual functioning (Schooler & Mulatu, 2001), we focused on all those respondents who provided data on their leisure-time activities and intellectual functioning. The effective sample size for this study was 635: 315 men and 320 women. They ranged in age from 41 to 88 years with a mean of 64.5. During the 1994-1995 follow-up interview, 265 (41.7%) were working for pay.

Substantive Complexity of Work

Substantively complex work was defined as work that in its very substance requires thought and independent judgment (Kohn & Schooler, 1983, p. 106). Indices for the latent concept of substantive complexity of work are derived from detailed open- and closed-ended questions about the participants' work with things, data (or ideas), and people. For the 1974 and 1994-1995 jobs, these questions provided the basis for seven ratings: appraisals of complexity of work with things, with data, and with people based on the ratings of complexity of work with things, data, and people in the *Dictionary of Occupational Titles* (United States Department of Labor, 1965); the respondents' estimates of the amount of time they spent working at each type of activity; and an appraisal of the overall complexity of work. Each index of complexity of work was rated on Likert-type scales. For example, complexity of work with data was rated on a 1 to 9 scale: 1 = no significant work with data to 9 = synthesizing. Hours of work with things ranged from 0 to 90 and were recorded as given.

Complexity of Leisure Activities

The cognitive complexity of leisure-time activities was conceptualized analogously to the complexity of paid work, except that the term refers to activities that are not done as part of paid work or housework. Our Cognitive Leisure Activities latent factor was measured by six items that were included in both the 1974 and 1994-1995 surveys. These were (1) the number of books read within the past six months; (2) the number of magazines read regularly; (2) the intellectual level of the magazines read, rated from low to high intellectuality on a 5-point scale; (4) the frequency of visits to fine art institutions or events including museums, concerts, and plays within the past six months; (5) the number of special interests, hobbies, and activities; and (6) the number of hours spent on special interests or hobbies.

Intellectual Flexibility

Intellectual Flexibility, the measure of intellectual functioning, is defined as cognitive flexibility in coping with the intellectual demands of a complex situation (see Kohn & Schooler, 1983, p. 112). Indices for this factor included the following: (1) a summary score for performance on a portion of the Embedded Figures Test (Witkin et al., 1962); (2) the interviewer's appraisal of the participant's intelligence made on the basis of the interviewer's impression during the interview session; (3) the frequency with which the respondent agreed when asked the many agree–disagree questions included in the interview (because some of the questions included in the battery were stated positively and others negatively, an overall tendency to agree suggested that the participant was not thinking carefully about and was less differentiating with regard to the questions); (4) a rating of the degree to which the answer to the question "What are all of the arguments you can think of for or against allowing cigarette commercials on TV?" provided reasons for both sides of the argument; and (5) a rating of the adequacy of the answer to a hypothetical question about how the respondent would decide between two alternate locations for a hamburger stand (adequacy being judged by a concern with potential costs and potential sales, as well as the understanding that profits result from the difference between the two).

The measures of Cognitive Leisure Activities and Intellectual Flexibility are strongly correlated with standard measures used elsewhere. Evidence that this is the case was found through correlating these factors with corresponding factors created with data from more standard measures available only in 1994-1995. Besides the six items used to indicate our longitudinal Cognitive Leisure Activity factor, the 1994-1995 data included five ratings of the complexity of tasks carried out with people and data and the hours spent on these activities that paralleled the measures of the substantive complexity of paid work. The correlation between SEM factors based on the two sets of items was quite high ($r = .89$, $p < .0001$). Similarly, the Intellectual Flexibility measure was highly correlated ($r = .86$, $p < .0001$) with a new factor based on standard cognitive tests, including immediate recall, category fluency, number series, verbal meaning, identical pictures, and different-uses tests. Thus, we confirmed that our survey-based intellectual functioning measure was as good a measure as the standard cognitive measures available in the field.

Data Analysis and Major Findings

Our general model showing the hypothesized reciprocal relationships between environmental complexity and intellectual functioning is shown in figure 2.1.

Job Complexity and Intellectual Functioning

In order to deal with the small sample size we had for this analysis (N = 233), we followed a two-stage causal modeling approach. Initially, a

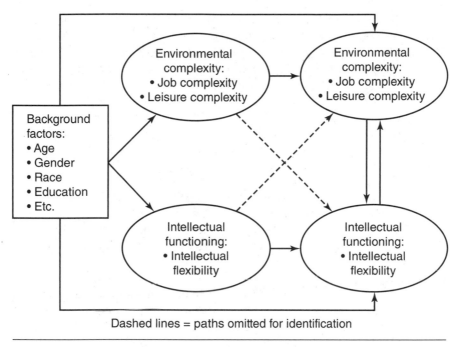

Dashed lines = paths omitted for identification

Figure 2.1 General model of reciprocal relationships.

measurement model was developed and estimated. This measurement model included not only the multi-indicator–based measures of Intellectual Flexibility and Substantive Complexity of Work, but also the single indicator–based measures of the background variables. The covariances between these measures were then saved and used as input data in the subsequent causal modeling. The model specifications were as follows: reciprocal effects between 1994-1995 Substantive Complexity of Work and 1994-1995 Intellectual Flexibility; paths from 1974 Substantive Complexity of Work and from 1974 Intellectual Flexibility to the corresponding 1994-1995 endogenous factors; and paths to these endogenous factors from all sociodemographic characteristics, including age, gender, education, and other demographic characteristics (included as statistical controls). Given our interest in age-related differences and similarities, we tested this model in an age-based multigroup analysis by splitting the sample into two age groups using the median age of 57. In testing this causal model, only the error and residual variances and covariances were allowed to vary across groups, and modification indices were inspected to determine the presence or absence of significant causal parameters that needed relaxing. In subsequent reestimations of the model, we also dropped insignificant structural paths.

Our final model fit the data very well, and the hypothesized relationships were confirmed. First, we found a significant path from 1994-1995 Substantive Complexity of Work to 1994-1995 Intellectual Flexibility, as well as a significant reverse path from 1994-1995 Intellectual Flexibility to 1994-1995 Substantive Complexity of Work—thus confirming the existence of reciprocal relationships. Second, we found a significant age-group difference in the path from 1994-1995 Substantive Complexity of Work to 1994-1995 Intellectual Flexibility, showing that the impact of Substantive Complexity on Intellectual Flexibility is about twice as great in the older group ($\beta = 0.50$, t = 14.87) as in the younger group ($\beta = 0.26$, t = 3.47). Third, although there was no age-group difference in the reverse path from 1994-1995 Intellectual Flexibility to 1994-1995 Substantive Complexity of Work, the relative magnitude of this path ($\beta = 0.25$) compared to its reciprocal (the path from 1994-1995 Substantive Complexity to 1994-1995 Intellectual Flexibility) was different for the two groups. For the younger group it was about the same size as the reciprocal effect of Substantive Complexity on Intellectual Flexibility; for the older group, it was about half the size. Generally similar results were obtained in a series of models that included a more extensive latent measure of the cognitive demands of paid work (i.e., Occupational Self-Direction) and full-information SEM (Schooler, Mulatu, & Oates, 2004).

Leisure Complexity and Intellectual Functioning

In contrast to our original analyses involving substantive complexity of paid work and intellectual flexibility (Schooler, Mulatu, & Oates, 1999), we used a full-information modeling approach in our analysis of the relationship between leisure-time activities and intellectual flexibility. The decisive factor was the relatively large sample size (N = 635) we have for handling our complex model. We also chose to compare the 1994-1995 working versus not working group, primarily because we believed that the nature and complexity of leisure-time activities are significantly associated with whether or not the individuals are working.

Having confirmed the validity of an invariant measurement model for our latent factors among working and nonworking groups and across the two time periods, we proposed the following causal parameters: (1) reciprocal effects between 1994-1995 Cognitive Leisure Activities and 1994-1995 Intellectual Flexibility, (2) paths from 1974 Cognitive Leisure Activities and 1974 Intellectual Flexibility to corresponding 1994-1995 endogenous factors, and (3) paths to 1994-1995 endogenous factors from all sociodemographic characteristics. In this model, only the error and residual variances and covariances were allowed to vary across groups, and modification indices were inspected to determine the presence or absence of significant causal parameters that needed relaxing. In subsequent reestimations of the model, we also dropped insignificant structural paths.

Our final model showed very good fit to the data (χ^2 [614, N = 635] = 1080.41; root-mean-square error of approximation, RMSEA = .05; comparative-fit index, CFI = .91), and also indicates that there were significant reciprocal effects between 1994-1995 Cognitive Leisure Activities and 1994-1995 Intellectual Flexibility. Being intellectually flexible resulted in carrying out relatively complex leisure activities (β = 0.34, $p \le$ .001). Conversely, carrying out relatively complex leisure activities resulted in higher levels of intellectual functioning (β = 0.26, $p \le$ .05). The effect of level of intellectual functioning on complexity of leisure-time activities was, in fact, slightly greater than the reciprocal effect. In this model, as in our model involving substantive complexity, background factors such as age, race, and socioeconomic status had both direct and indirect effects on Cognitive Leisure Activities and Intellectual Flexibility. The reciprocal relationship between cognitive leisure activities and intellectual functioning remained even after employment status was taken into account using multigroup analyses that examined the working and nonworking respondents separately.

Significance of the Findings

The pattern of our findings indicates that the cognitive complexity of both the paid work and the leisure-time activities of middle-aged and older adults affects their intellectual functioning. Doing more complex work and leisure-time activities increases intellectual functioning; doing less complex work or leisure activities decreases intellectual functioning. As we have seen, this causal pattern holds true when we compare the effects of complex paid work on older and younger workers and of complex leisure-time activities on older and younger individuals. The effects of complex leisure-time activities are also the same for those who work for pay and those who do not. We have also found evidence that the reciprocal effect exists. Having higher levels of intellectual functioning leads people to carry out more complex paid work as well as more intellectually demanding leisure-time activities. Although the reciprocal effects we found are relatively modest, they indicate that the intellectual benefits for middle-aged and older adults of doing intellectually challenging things on the job and off the job are significant and meaningful.

Our results extend Kohn and Schooler's earlier (1983) findings about the effects of substantive complexity of work on intellectual functioning when the present sample was 20 years younger. Our findings also indicate that the effects of dealing with cognitively complex environmental demands on the cognitive functioning of both the older and younger members of our sample extend beyond doing such work for pay to carrying out relatively cognitively complex leisure-time tasks. Together, our findings about work and leisure time provide consistent, credibly strong evidence that even in old age, carrying out self-directed complex tasks has a positive effect on intellectual processes. They thus afford further support for the generalizability of the hypothesis (Schooler, 1984, 1990) that dealing with cognitively demanding environments increases one's level of intellectual functioning throughout the life span. Within the age range of our sample (41-88 years), the effects of environmental conditions on psychological functioning are at least as strong for older as for younger adults. Indeed, in one of the studies, we found greater effects of substantive complexity on intellectual functioning in older than in younger adults, suggesting that older adults may be psychologically more affected by environmental conditions than younger ones. These findings raise the practical issues of the desirability and possibility of societal interventions to at least maintain the complexity of the environments to which older individuals are exposed.

All in all, our findings strongly suggest that, even if doing crossword puzzles per se may not be effective (cf. Hambrick, Salthouse, & Meinz, 1999), doing substantively complex tasks, either at work or at leisure, is an "analog of aerobic exercises" (Hertzog, Hultsch, & Dixon, 1999, p. 528). Even in old age, working out on a regimen of substantively complex tasks appears to build the capacity to deal with the intellectual challenges that complex environments provide.

Human (Quasi-) Experimental Studies on Environmental Complexity and Intellectual Functioning

The SSES findings, however, are primarily based on longitudinal survey data. As such, they do not pretend to explicate the basic neurobiological or psychosocial mechanisms through which complex environments and intellectual functioning affect one another. There have, of course, been many experimental animal studies dealing with relevant psychoneurobiologial issues that chapters in this volume will address (for a comprehensive recent review see Mohammed et al., 2002), so I will not discuss them here. Instead, I briefly review some quasi-experimental human intervention studies that not only provide supporting evidence for the cognitive effects of exposure to complex environments, but also suggest potential neurobiological and psychological mechanisms through which exposure to cognitively complex environments affects intellectual functioning.

Spector and colleagues (2003) conducted a randomized controlled trial to evaluate the efficacy of an evidence-based cognitive stimulation program on cognitive functioning and quality of life of people with dementia. The intervention group received 14 sessions (45 min per session) of cognitive stimulation and reality orientation, focusing on such topics as using money, word games, present day, famous faces, and a range of other personal and social activities. Compared to the control group participants who did not participate in these sessions, intervention participants showed significant improvement in their cognitive functioning as well as in their quality of life. The authors noted that the magnitude of the intervention effects were comparable to those reported in clinical trials of drugs for dementia.

Ball and colleagues (2002) conducted a larger and more elaborate randomized controlled trial to evaluate the effectiveness of three forms of cognitive training interventions in improving cognitive and daily functioning in independent-living older adults. The three intervention groups received 10 sessions (60-75 min per session) of training in verbal episodic memory, problem-solving reasoning, and speed of processing, respectively. The intervention sessions involved instructions on cognitive strategies with increasing difficulty levels as well as individual and group exercises to practice these strategies. Booster sessions were provided after 11 months of the initial intervention for 60% of the original participants. The study revealed that each intervention improved the targeted cognitive ability compared to the baseline and control group values both on the immediate posttraining evaluation and, to a lesser extent, on the second evaluation at 24 months. Unlike Spector and colleagues (2003), Ball's group did not find that the positive effects of cognitive training significantly generalized to improvement in everyday functioning. An earlier experimental training study by Willis and Schaie (1986), however, does provide proof that training older adults can yield generalization across cognitive skills demonstrated by SEM to belong to different latent factors.

Conclusions

Mohammed and colleagues (2002) summarize their recent extensive review of neurobiological research on environmental enrichment and the brain by noting that "the findings of environmentally induced changes in the brains of aged organisms are compatible with the notion of 'use it or lose it'" (p. 126). They conclude by asserting that "environmental stimulation can sustain neurotrophin levels in this [i.e., basal forebrain] and other brain regions and help to maintain function by increasing neural reserve in the aged individual. The impact of environmental enrichment on the brain appears to be a universal phenomenon having been observed in many different species—from flies to philosophers" (p. 127). This survey of relevant psychological and sociological research on the effects of cognitively complex environments on human intellectual functioning provides quite consistent support for this point of view from the behavioral sciences. The results of SEM-based reciprocal-effects models demonstrate that the correlations found between levels of intellectual functioning and environmental complexity are due, at least in part, to such environmental effects. These analyses very substantially reduce the possibility that such correlations result solely from the degree to which individuals who function well intellectually select or are selected into cognitively demanding environments and are more able to successfully maintain themselves in such conditions than those functioning less well intellectually.

Finally, although, as we have seen, both our own and others' findings quite consistently support the hypotheses that engaging in cognitively demanding activities, both on and off of the job, has a positive effect on intellectual functioning, at present we have at best an only rudimentary idea of the psychological and neurobiological processes underlying such an effect. Furthermore, we have no real idea of what the limits of such environmental effects on cognitive functioning are and how such limits may change during different stages of the life course. Nevertheless, everything we know points to the fact that the intellectual functioning of older individuals benefits from their dealing with the cognitive challenges presented by relatively complex environments. At least for some, using "it" helps in not losing "it."

CHAPTER 3

Enhancing Cognitive Function in Older Adults

Michelle L. Meade
Department of Psychology, Montana State University

Denise C. Park, PhD
School of Behavioral and Brain Sciences, University of Texas at Dallas

It is well established that aging is accompanied by cognitive decline, and there is currently great interest in understanding contextual moderators of such decline. Improving cognitive function in older adults, even by a small amount, has important consequences for older adults' quality of life, particularly if enhancements defer the age at which susceptible adults become disabled due to Alzheimer's disease. The current chapter provides a discussion of two approaches aimed at improving cognitive function in older adults. One approach is based on laboratory interventions in which subjects are trained in an effort to improve specific cognitive functions, and the other approach focuses on the role that lifestyle variables might play in preserving cognitive function in older adults. After a brief overview of cognitive aging, we discuss the two approaches in turn, giving emphasis to the overall effectiveness of each. Finally, we discuss new research involving experimental manipulation of lifestyle variables that we believe offers promising new directions for aging interventions.

Overview of Cognitive Aging

Compelling evidence exists that with age, there are reliable declines in information-processing speed (Salthouse, 1996); working memory capacity (Park et al., 1996, 2002); the ability to task-switch or inhibit irrelevant information (Cepeda et al., 2001; Hasher & Zacks, 1979); and long-term memory function, especially encoding (Craik, 1983; Park et al., 1996, 2002). In addition to the processing declines, there is also evidence that accrued knowledge (which represents the effects of experience) improves with age. The interaction between processing decline and knowledge growth is represented in figure 3.1 (Park et al., 2002).

Of interest is the impact that simultaneous processing decline and increased knowledge have on older adults' cognitive function. Recent

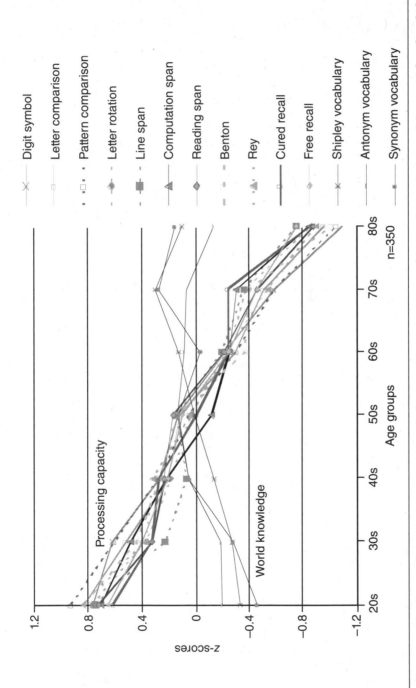

Figure 3.1 Life span performance measures: speed of processing measures, working memory measures (visuospatial and verbal), long-term memory measures (visuospatial and verbal), short-term memory measures (visuospatial and verbal), and knowledge-based verbal ability measures. Composite scores for each construct represent the z score of the average of all measures for that construct.

Reprinted from D.L. Park et al., 2002. "Models of visuospatial and verbal memory across the adult life span," *Psychology and Aging* 17(2): 299-320. By permission of D.C. Park.

research suggests that increased knowledge may exert a protective effect on cognition, as older adults may rely on this increased knowledge to compensate for processing deficits. For example, Hedden, Lautenschlager, and Park (2005), using structural equation modeling, reported that older adults relied more on verbal knowledge to remember paired associates and produce words in a verbal fluency task while younger adults relied more on speed of processing and working memory capacity.

Along with evidence of age-related decreases in behavioral processes, there is also evidence that many neural structures shrink with age. Frontal lobe volume has been shown to decrease across the life span, and more moderate shrinkage has been observed in the medial temporal areas (Raz, 2000). Short-term longitudinal studies have indicated that volumetric changes in brain structure are evident in healthy older adults after only a single year. Specifically, healthy older adults in the Baltimore Longitudinal Study demonstrated brain volume decreases (in both gray and white matter) of an average of 5.4 cm^3 per year (Resnick et al., 2003) and also reliable increases in ventricular volume (fluid-filled areas that increase as the brain shrinks) (Resnick et al., 2000).

Despite the decrease in neural tissue with age, it is typically the case that in functional neuroimaging studies, older adults show greater distribution of activation across brain sites than young adults during encoding and working memory tasks, and most frequently show increased or bilateral activation in prefrontal areas when young adults show unilateral activation (Cabeza, 2002; Park et al., 2003; Reuter-Lorenz, 2002). Considerable theorizing suggests that this additional activation in the older adults may be compensatory for a declining neural system (Cabeza, 2002; Park et al., 2001; Daselaar et al., 2003; Rosen et al., 2002). In support of this hypothesis, Gutchess and colleagues (2005) reported that older adults utilized more middle frontal cortex than younger subjects to encode pictures they later remembered, whereas young adults relied more on hippocampal activations. Moreover, there was a direct relationship between increased frontal and decreased hippocampal activations in old but not young subjects. This pattern of findings suggests that older adults compensated for hippocampal processing deficits by recruiting additional resources from the frontal areas.

Evidence from neuroimaging studies strongly suggests that older adults may compensate for decline by recruiting different or additional neural areas (or both). The flexibility inherent in this compensation suggests that older adults' neural function is dynamic and that plasticity remains in the neurocognitive system in late adulthood. Moreover, a limited behavioral literature indicates that older adults utilize different and often efficient strategies to compensate for declining cognition (e.g., Hedden, Lautenschlager, & Park, 2005; Hertzog, Dunlosky, & Robinson, 2005b). This reorganization and adaptation is the focus of this chapter. We are interested in understanding ways in which cognitive decline in older adults can be attenuated, and we devote the remainder of the chapter to intervention strategies for improving cognition in late adulthood. We focus the discussion on intervention programs conducted in the laboratory, as well as lifestyle variables and potential interventions that may enhance cognitive function. There is also a large literature on external variables and cues (such as semantic relationships, supportive visual stimuli, list organization) designed to support rather than change cognitive function with age, but we do not consider such stimulus-specific manipulations in this chapter.

Laboratory-Based Studies of Active Cognitive Facilitation

Perhaps the most commonly used laboratory technique designed to enhance cognitive function in older adults is training. In a typical training study, older adults are trained on a specific cognitive task or process in which cognitive decline is evident, with the aim of examining any potential improvement on related tasks. For example, if individuals were trained in a name–face memory technique, one might expect improvement in their ability to remember names and faces at a cocktail party, as this task would be very similar to their original training (evidence for near transfer). Of further interest in training studies is whether improvement on the trained task transfers to improvement on novel tasks, for example whether a name–face training technique improves working memory function or driving (far transfer). The idea is that the sustained exercise of a particular mental process may strengthen cognitive function in a variety of domains, much as physical exercise will result in an increase in strength in the specific muscles exercised as well as general improvements in overall fitness and cardiovascular capacity.

Willis and Schaie (1986) provide evidence that training is effective for improving cognitive function in a specific domain and also stabilizing declining cognitive function. Older adults in this study were classified, according to data collected longitudinally over the prior 14 years, as either stable or as evidencing decline on spatial orientation and inductive reasoning abilities. All subjects received five training sessions on either spatial orientation or inductive reasoning over a two-week period. Using a construct-based approach to measure change, Willis and Schaie reported significant improvements in both inductive reasoning and spatial orientation as a function of training. More importantly, training stabilized performance for subjects who had previously demonstrated decline on the target abilities, and it improved performance for subjects whose performance had remained stable. The results suggest that training selectively improved cognitive function, but there was no evidence for general strengthening (note that training did not transfer to novel tasks—subjects in the spatial orientation condition did not improve in inductive reasoning or vice versa).

In perhaps the most comprehensive training study conducted to date, Ball and colleagues (2002) enrolled 2800 subjects in training programs for memory function, speed of processing, or reasoning. Subjects were trained over a six-week period and received 10 one-hour training sessions overall; a subset also received additional booster training 11 months later. Subjects were given an immediate performance test as well as yearly follow-up evaluations for two successive years. Of interest was the impact of training on the target abilities (memory, speed of processing, and reasoning), but also the impact of training on activities of daily living such as food preparation and financial management (these activities were measured on the Instrumental Activities of Daily Living Scale [IADL], e.g., Willis et al., 1992). Ball and colleagues hypothesized that since memory, speed of processing, and reasoning were involved in successful execution of daily living tasks, improving these component processes should transfer to an improvement in daily living scores. Results indicated that the training improved older adults' performance on the domain in which they were trained, but there was no transfer to improvement on tasks of everyday living. Moreover, consistent with much prior research on training, Ball and colleagues showed benefits of training on the specific ability trained, but no transfer to novel tasks.

Subjects in the studies by Willis and Schaie (1986) and Ball and colleagues (2002) were classified as healthy older adults. An interesting question concerns the effectiveness of stabilizing cognitive abilities in older adults with memory problems. Cherry and Simmons-D'Gerolamo (2005) provided memory training to older adults with probable Alzheimer's disease. Using a spaced-retrieval program in which progressively longer intervals interspersed successful retrieval, the authors demonstrated reliable improvements on immediate tests. Long-term effects of spaced retrieval on memory performance of probable Alzheimer's patients are difficult to obtain (Cherry & Simmons-D'Gerolamo, 1999), although those trained previously showed an advantage on retraining trials (Cherry & Simmons-D'Gerolamo, 2005). The immediate improvement suggests that training may in some cases affect even cognitively impaired older adults (see Camp et al., 1996, 2000 and Cherry & Smith, 1998 for reviews).

Most recently the impact of training on neural structures has been examined. Relatively few studies in older adults have addressed whether cognitive training can result in a permanent change in neural structure or function, although there is evidence that changes can occur in young adults. For example, Draganski and colleagues (2004) trained young adults on a simple juggling routine over a period of three months and found that sustained juggling increased gray matter in the midtemporal area and the left posterior intraparietal sulcus. In a study that involved both young and older adults, Nyberg and colleagues (2003) demonstrated that mnemonic training increased frontal and occipitoparietal activation in young adults. Older adults also demonstrated neural plasticity, but the pattern was different. Only those older adults whose memory improved with the mnemonic showed increased occipitoparietal activation, and none of the older adults increased frontal activations. Other evidence of plasticity with age comes from work by Colcombe and colleagues (2003), who reported that older subjects who improved aerobic fitness showed more gray matter in the frontal, temporal, and parietal regions compared to sedentary older adults. Although relatively sparse at this time, evidence that training permanently increases neural volume or changes neural circuitry for a sustained period will be important in future training work to demonstrate efficacy.

Training provides a relatively effective means of improving cognitive function on the target ability (near transfer) and in some cases has important implications for quality of life (as in memory training for older adults with probable Alzheimer's disease, or training older adults on techniques that will increase their medication adherence), but important limitations exist in the majority of training studies. As outlined by Marsiske (2005), any improvement from training is relatively short-lived, and not all subjects are able to benefit from training. Marsiske also addressed perhaps the biggest challenge facing training studies: demonstrating far transfer. That is, improving or stabilizing a single target ability does not transfer to improvement in other single abilities, let alone to a more global cognitive improvement such that older adults might benefit in domains outside of laboratory tasks. One exception is training the useful field of view (UFOV), which may transfer to better driving ability in older adults (Roenker et al., 2003).

Training studies typically involve sustained practice over a number of days as a mechanism for improving or strengthening cognitive function. Virtually all of the training literature relies on repetition of effortful, top-down cognitive processes that have declined with age, on the assumption that repeated performance of the process will make the operation easier or more efficient to perform on a range of tasks. Another approach to improving cognitive function relies on exploiting cognitive processes that are age invariant and do not decline with age (Park, 2000). Such automatic processes (Hasher & Zacks, 1979) utilize few cognitive resources and tend to be bottom-up, data-driven processes that are activated in response to environmental cues or suggestions. Because such automatic processes are particularly sensitive to the environment, they may be useful for enhancing cognitive performance in real-world situations, such as remembering to take medications or implement medical procedures.

Liu and Park (2004) relied on activation of automatic processes to improve medical adherence in older adults. They instructed older subjects in the use of a glucose monitor and then indicated that the subjects should monitor their glucose four times a day at specific times for the next three weeks. Subjects were assigned to a condition in which they actively rehearsed the intention (engaging an effortful process) or one in which they deliberated about pros and cons associated with the action (also effortful). In a third condition, subjects formed "implementation intentions," which involved imagining performance of the glucose-monitoring behavior in the specific context they expected to be in at the target time on the next day. For example, they might imagine themselves drinking orange juice with breakfast and then monitoring their blood glucose after they drank the juice at the appointed time. When they actually drank their orange juice the following morning, this act would automatically cue them to also monitor their blood glucose level. This reliance on automatic processes to enhance adherence yielded clear evidence that the implementation training (which took 5 min) increased use of the glucose monitor at the appointed times relative to the other two conditions. Remarkably, this significant increase was maintained for the entire three weeks of the study. Liu and Park suggested that because the older adults led relatively routine lives, once they implemented the behavior they tended to encounter the same cues in their environment each day, which continued to stimulate and maintain the glucose monitoring. These data suggest that another effective technique for improving cognitive function may involve capitalizing on intact automatic processes in older adults as a mechanism for improving function in different situations.

Lifestyle Variables as Predictors of Late-Life Cognitive Function

In light of the facts that training older adults on specific cognitive abilities does little to improve overall cognitive function, and that reliance on automatic processes is necessarily limited to particular situations, it is important to examine other means by which cognition may be enhanced in older adults. One approach is to examine lifestyle variables. There is some evidence that sustained involvement of various cognitive functions across the life span favorably affects cognitive function in late adulthood. Further, because the activities in real life may be more varied and complex than activities trained in the laboratory, benefit from sustained participation in these activities could be more likely to be supportive of a broad array of cognitive functions.

Research on lifestyle variables assesses cognitive function between groups of people who have been more or less engaged in particular types of activities throughout their lives. Of interest is whether those individuals who have been more active in a given activity demonstrate higher cognitive function than individuals who have not been active in that activity.

Lifestyle research is largely correlational, leading to interpretive issues (see Salthouse, in press for a discussion). However, the effects are powerful, and across many studies the correlation exists between leading an engaged life and exhibiting higher cognitive function. Evidence that lifestyle variables influence the rate of cognitive decline in older adults comes from literature on intellectual engagement in complex work and cognitive activities, engagement in leisure activities, and social engagement. We next review each in turn.

One approach to understanding the effect of lifestyle variables on later cognition is to examine the cognitive health of older adults who have spent a lifetime employed in complex jobs relative to individuals who have spent a lifetime employed in less complex jobs. Many years of engaging in the cognitive effort required for complex jobs may exert a protective benefit against later cognitive decline. The evidence concerning whether intellectually challenging environments favorably influence cognition during late adulthood is mixed. Many studies support the hypothesis that cognitively demanding work environments foster greater cognitive function in old age. For example, Schooler and colleagues (1999) reported that engagement in "substantively complex" work across the life span predicted better intellectual functioning in old age than did engagement in less challenging work, even after education and other related factors were controlled. Schooler and colleagues proposed a reciprocal model suggesting that people who have higher cognitive function are more likely to engage in activities and that these activities foster higher cognitive function—so that there is a feedback loop maintaining higher cognitive function in active older adults. Further evidence showing that complex work may protect against cognitive decline comes from the Maastricht Longitudinal Study. None of the participants showed cognitive impairment at the beginning of the study; but three years later, 4% of those with jobs that imposed low cognitive demands showed some cognitive impairment, whereas only 1.5% of those with mentally demanding jobs were impaired (Bosma et al., 2003).

Other studies, however, are mixed in relation to the hypothesis that complex work helps maintain cognitive function in late adulthood. Shimamura and colleagues (1995) compared age effects between young and older professors to age effects between undergraduates and community-dwelling older adults. While professors demonstrated age deficits comparable to those of the general population on measures of reaction time, paired-associate learning, and working memory, they demonstrated no age effects on measures of proactive interference and prose recall, in contrast to the general population, who did demonstrate age effects. Likewise, research by Christensen (1994) suggests that age differences between young and older professors are reduced on some but not all tests of memory relative to age effects observed for young and old manual laborers.

Finally, evidence exists to refute the claim that demanding work spares cognitive processes. Christensen and colleagues (1997) showed that professors and blue-collar workers did not differ in their rate of decline on nonverbal tasks across a five-year longitudinal study. Further, Salthouse and colleagues (1990) showed that architects were no better on visual-spatial tasks than were nonarchitects—evidence that seemingly contradicts the hypothesis that demanding work facilitates cognitive function.

Possible explanations for the mixed findings regarding quality of work experience and cognition in late adulthood may be related to the definition of a complex job. Operational definitions for complex work vary widely in the literature just cited, which deals with jobs ranging from blue collar versus white collar (Christensen et al., 1997) to nonprofessor versus professor (Shimamura et al., 1995). Further, individuals vary in terms of how intellectually invested they are in a given profession. For example, some professors frequently update class material to include challenging new information while others simply repeat the same class material for several years in a row. Finally, the effects of work experience may be small and may become apparent only at very old age, such that a lifetime of complex work may provide subtle protective effects that are not readily measured.

Another potential way to examine the impact of engagement is to consider how engaged people are within a given profession. Despite concerns about self-report, examining self-reported level of cognitive engagement better addresses the wide individual differences between people of similar occupational status. The literature suggests that individuals' self-reported involvement in cognitive activities does have a relationship to cognitive function in later life. Specifically, Wilson and colleagues asked subjects to rate their level of involvement in a variety of cognitively demanding activities ranging from watching television to listening to the radio, reading, playing games, and visiting museums. Individuals who self-reported greater involvement in these activities performed better on a cognitive battery (Wilson et al., 1999, 2003) and showed reduced risk of Alzheimer's disease (Wilson, Mendes de Leon et al., 2002; Wilson, Bennett et al., 2002) relative to individuals who self-reported less involvement in those activities. The results of these studies are quite remarkable, as they include extremely large and diverse samples and suggest that even a slight increase in cognitive activities can reduce the risk of dementia by as much as 64% (Wilson, Bennett et al., 2002).

Further, individuals who self-report higher levels of participation in cognitively demanding activities have been shown to perform better on laboratory measures of memory. Arbuckle and colleagues (1992) found a small, independent effect for self-reported engagement in intellectual activities across the life span on multiple measures of memory in a sample of World War II veterans, although general intelligence predicted the most variance. In a later study on this sample, Pushkar Gold and colleagues (1995) suggested that initially high levels of intellectual ability and education conferred both the inclination and opportunity to develop an engaged lifestyle, which in turn conferred additional benefits on cognition in late adulthood. This idea is similar to the reciprocal model of Schooler and colleagues (1999) discussed previously and represents a fundamental issue in understanding the influence of lifestyle variables on cognitive function. Does intellectual activity enhance cognitive function, or is it that those individuals with initially higher levels of cognitive function are more active in intellectually engaging activities? The interpretive issues inherent in this discussion are exemplified in data reported by Hultsch and colleagues (1999). These authors found that individuals in the Victoria Longitudinal Study who self-reported high levels of engagement in intellectual activities across six years were buffered from cognitive decline. However, according to the authors, another explanation for the data could be that individuals with high cognitive functioning seek out intellectually engaging activities. Further experimental research is needed to better understand possible mechanisms underlying the correlational evidence. In general, it appears that self-reported engagement in cognitive activities is related to higher cognitive function across the life span.

Note that these studies used a composite measure of multiple cognitive constructs. Research on the effect of self-reported involvement in a single cognitive activity often does not show significant benefits. For example, Hambrick and coworkers (1999) found that individuals who self-reported greater experience with crossword puzzles did no better on a cognitive battery than those who reported low levels of crossword experience (for related findings see Salthouse & Mitchell, 1990; Salthouse et al., 2002). The difference between findings of self-reported engagement in single activities (e.g., crossword puzzles) and self-reported engagement in a range of cognitively engaging activities (e.g., radio, television, museums) may reflect an underlying level of general activity. Similar to what is suggested by the reciprocal model outlined earlier, individuals who self-report higher levels of engagement across activities might be generally more active and thus seek out more challenging activities that feed back to increasing cognitive function. In contrast, individuals who self-report mastery of a single skill might not transfer that skill to novel areas and thus may not derive the same benefits as people who are more broadly engaged in cognitively demanding activities. Nonetheless, the research provides insight into whether intellectual engagement offers a protective effect on late-life cognitive function and the role of intellectual engagement in later life.

Several studies have explored the possible impact of leisure activities on older adults' cognitive function. The underlying assumption in these studies is that participating in leisure activities exercises a variety of skills that may later buffer cognitive decline. Fabrigoule and colleagues (1995[N]) reported that traveling, gardening, and knitting offered a protective effect against developing dementia for older adults tested within three years of baseline screening. Scarmea and colleagues (2001) found that individuals who self-reported engagement in a higher number of leisure activities (including visiting friends and walking) had a reduced risk of dementia even when initial cognitive performance, health, and depression were controlled for. Finally, Crowe and coworkers (2003) showed that the overall number of leisure activities (intellectual-cultural, domestic, and self-improvement) reported during early and middle adulthood was associated with lower risk of dementia in late adulthood. Note that leisure is difficult to measure, as leisure activities often entail cognitive, social, and physical components (see Kramer et al., 1999 and Colcombe & Kramer, 2003 for reviews of the beneficial effects of physical activity on cognition). Wang and colleagues (2002) provide evidence that leisure activities benefit cognition even when physical activity is adjusted for. Generally, compelling data suggest that leisure activities may benefit cognitive function in older adults by reducing risk of dementia, although it is not always clear which component process of leisure activities might be driving the effect.

Social Activities

There is a literature suggesting that a high degree of engagement in exclusively social activities is associated with enhanced cognitive functions in older adults. Social engagement is typically defined in terms of contact with others in the context of living situations (marital status, contact with children) and out-of-home activities (social activities with friends and family) and also in terms of satisfaction with social encounters. Although it may seem surprising, social encounters place a high demand on many aspects of cognitive function, particularly memory. Social appropriateness makes it important for people to remember names, and as a relationship with an acquaintance develops, to remember many elements of the person's life, family, and activities as the basis for further interactions. Barnes and coworkers (2004) demonstrated that having a greater number of social networks was correlated with higher cognitive function in older adults and also slowed the rate of cognitive decline. Further, social engagement may have a protective effect against developing dementia in old age (Seidler et al., 2003). In a longitudinal, population-based study in Sweden, risk of a dementia diagnosis was 60% greater in individuals with a limited social network (Fratiglioni et al., 2000). Similarly, Bassuk and colleagues (1999) reported a substantial increase in risk of cognitive impairment for individuals who had engaged in limited social activities 12 years earlier. These data suggest that people who maintain high levels of social support may demonstrate higher cognitive function (and a reduced risk of dementia) in later life. Keep in mind that the data discussed are correlational, so no directional relationships can be identified between social engagement (or other lifestyle variables) and cognitive function.

Summary

Many correlational studies suggest a relationship between lifestyle variables and cognitive function in old age. Further, in contrast to findings from the training studies discussed earlier in the chapter, lifestyle variables result in relatively more global cognitive improvements. Such research is promising and supports the notion that cognitive and neural circuitry are flexible even into late adulthood. One important issue that cannot be addressed by the current body of literature is the mechanism underlying these effects, and more specifically whether lifestyle variables are leading to higher cognition or whether higher-functioning older adults are those who are choosing lifestyle variables to maintain their heightened levels of cognitive function (see the reciprocal model proposed by Schooler et al., 1999). To really understand the impact of lifestyle variables on older adults' cognitive function, experimental research is needed in which older adults are randomly assigned to participate in intellectually engaging activities.

In two experimental studies, we have attempted to directly manipulate participation in stimulating activities to determine the influence of lifestyle variables on older adults' cognitive function. The stimulating activities chosen were learning to quilt and learning to use a digital camera. In both cases, subjects were randomly selected to be in the experimental group (in which they learned to quilt or use a digital camera) or a wait-list control group. All subjects received pretesting on a full cognitive battery. Subjects in the experimental group then participated in 15 hr per week of activities related to the intervention. Of these 15 hr each week, 5 hr were spent in structured classes and 10 hr were spent working on the techniques learned in class. The intervention lasted eight weeks, so overall the experimental subjects logged at least 120 hr of time engaging in the novel activity. In contrast, subjects in the control group were called once a week and asked about their daily activities. At the end of eight weeks, all subjects completed a posttest consisting of the same cognitive battery given at pretest. Finding selective improvement on the posttest for subjects in the experimental group relative to the control group would argue in support of the hypothesis that lifestyle interventions benefit cognitive function in older adults—that it is not simply that higher-functioning older adults are selecting challenging activities.

Preliminary results indicated that subjects who participated in the quilting intervention selectively improved on measures of speed of processing and that the digital camera participants showed selective improvements in long-term memory. Given the small number of subjects tested, combined with the difficulties often associated with getting substantial effect sizes for interactions, the results are promising and suggest that experimentally controlled intervention studies may yield useful information for understanding the role of lifestyle variables on cognitive function in older adults.

Future Directions

There are many unanswered questions about enhancing cognitive function in older adults. The research reviewed in the current chapter suggests that one of the most important questions facing the field involves identifying mechanisms responsible for cognitive flexibility so that interventions can be more effectively implemented. Experimental research on lifestyle variables provides a promising new approach for possibly disentangling the effects of activities from the initial cognitive function of the individuals. Future research might also focus more on the neural underpinnings of cognitive flexibility to provide a better understanding of the biological bases for cognitive change. Given the importance of intervention work for the daily lives of older adults, one final goal of future research might involve improving the implementation of interventions so that older adults might more easily benefit from this area of research.

CHAPTER 4

A Contextual Approach to Aging and Expertise

Daniel G. Morrow

Institute of Aviation,
University of Illinois at Urbana-Champaign

We hope to age gracefully, offsetting biological changes underlying loss of physical, sensory, and cognitive function with gains in knowledge, efficiency, and wisdom, the fruits of experience. Research both supports and limits this optimistic vision of aging, revealing complex trade-offs between age-related gains and losses that influence our ability to accomplish daily activities. Decades of laboratory research paint a somewhat pessimistic view, with age-graded declines on tasks requiring fluid mental abilities such as speeded processing, working memory, and reasoning necessitated by novel tasks (e.g., Park et al., 1996). However, research rooted in meaningful, familiar situations at work and home presents a more encouraging view. For example, age is often unrelated to performance on work tasks (e.g., Salthouse & Maurer, 1996). This discrepancy may reflect the fact that work and home activities often depend more on knowledge and skills garnered from experience than on fluid abilities. Such "crystallized abilities" tend to be maintained or even to increase across the life span, even as the rate of acquiring new knowledge slows (Ackerman & Rolfhus, 1999). Other aspects of "pragmatic intelligence" important to daily function, such as wisdom (Baltes & Staudinger, 1993) and social judgments (Hess, Osowski, & Leclerc, 2005), may also increase with age.

Not surprisingly, there is long-standing interest in understanding the extent to which older adults' competence is maintained by expertise, and in *how* this knowledge and experience offsets age-related cognitive declines (for reviews see Bosman & Charness, 1996; Rybash, Hoyer, & Roodin, 1987; Salthouse, 1990, 1995). These issues are especially pertinent today because of the recognition that cognition and aging must be studied in context (Stern & Carstensen, 2000) and because of interest in analyzing daily competence in terms of person–environment transactions, both in life span theory (e.g., Diehl, 1998; Lawton, 1982) and in human factors theory (e.g., distributed-cognition theories; Hutchins, 1995). More practical issues have also focused attention on expert–age relationships. Demographic, economic, and other societal changes have encouraged policy makers to revisit age-based retirement rules for pilots (Sirven & Morrow, 2007) and air traffic specialists (Broach & Schroeder, 2006). More generally, today's older adults will work more years than earlier generations, raising issues of benefits (and costs) of past experience for maintaining and learning new skills.

Overview

I first consider how experts excel on domain-relevant tasks despite cognitive limitations, which suggests ways in which older experts may offset age-related cognitive constraints to maintain performance. Expertise is not a single category: Experts excel in many different ways (Hoffman et al., 1995). Therefore, rather than ask whether expertise reduces age-related differences in performance, it is more useful to consider under what circumstances mitigation occurs. To do this, I adopt Jenkins' contextual framework for memory research (Jenkins, 1979) in order to explore how expertise (and expertise-based mitigation of age differences) depends on characteristics of person (e.g., level of expertise, cognitive abilities, age), task (e.g., difficulty, time pressure, domain relevance), and performance assessment (e.g., recall or reasoning). These characteristics may jointly influence the likelihood of experts' adopting strategies that mitigate age effects. Moreover, because expertise mechanisms may differ by domain, the chapter is organized into two broad areas: (a) domains in which performance depends heavily on perceptual and attentional skills that are highly adapted to rule-based constraints; and (b) more open-ended domains in which performance depends on complex cognitive skills such planning, situation awareness, and task management. The latter domains may allow a greater repertoire of strategies that mitigate age-related differences in fluid mental abilities (Rybash, Hoyer, & Roodin, 1986).

Expertise and Cognitive Efficiency

Experts do not appear to excel because of superior general cognitive abilities (which could occur because they were initially selected or later retained based on these abilities, or because experience honed the abilities): Experts and novices typically do not differ on measures of processing speed, working memory, or other general cognitive abilities; and the two groups tend to experience similar age-related changes in general cognitive abilities (e.g., Clancy & Hoyer, 1994; Morrow et al., 2003). Rather, expertise benefits hinge on the extent to which tasks embody domain-relevant constraints, as shown by the finding that expertise-related benefits are reduced as these constraints are eliminated (for review see Vicente & Wang, 1998). Thus, expert performance depends on highly organized knowledge structures in long-term memory that enable experts to view problems at an abstract level (Glaser & Chi, 1988).

By exploiting this domain knowledge, experts efficiently accomplish task goals in several ways. First, efficient attentional strategies such as focusing on the most problem-relevant information are guided by abstract problem representations (Bellenkes, Wickens, & Kramer, 1997; Shanteau, 1992). Second, efficiency is gained because knowledge reduces the need for cognitively intensive computations (Feignbaum, 1989). Experts also develop complex retrieval structures that enable rapid and reliable access to these knowledge structures in long-term memory, thus bypassing to some extent working memory capacity limitations (long-term working memory; Ericsson & Kintsch, 1995). Third, high levels of experience on domain-relevant tasks can automatize perceptual-motor skills, reducing dependency on limited attentional resources (Anderson, 1990). Finally, experts excel through external as well as internal (mental) strategies. They reduce cognitive complexity by interacting with their environment so as to offload mental workload onto external forms of cognition (Hutchins, 1995; Kirlik, 1995).

To sum up, experts achieve high levels of performance through a variety of strategies that have the potential to offset age-related cognitive declines and maintain performance. These strategies roughly correspond to mechanisms identified as underlying expert-based mitigation (e.g., Bosman & Charness, 1996; Salthouse, 1990). Older experts may engage in high levels of practice that support efficient skills (skill maintenance); they may develop new strategies to offset recognized age-related cognitive declines, such as increasingly focusing on the most relevant information, relying on external aids, or relying on collaborative relationships (compensation); or they may simplify tasks so as to reduce cognitive demands of accomplishing them (accommodation). The following sections identify person, task, and performance assessment conditions that influence when these strategies are adopted.

Before we review these studies, it is worth noting that they vary in design and thus in how evidence for mitigation is evaluated. Some studies use extreme-groups designs to test age $\times$ expertise interactions (reduced age effects for more expert groups). Other studies use samples in which age and experience vary continuously, with age and expertise effects tested in regression models. Small samples often limit the ability of studies with either design to detect key relationships between age and expertise. Another common methodological challenge lies in the fact that experience tends to increase with age (a "confound of nature"). Regression analyses are sometimes used to evaluate whether age-related variance in performance increases when experience differences are controlled, suggesting that experience buffers the effects of age among those with more experience (Meinz, 2000). Other studies use a longitudinal design to examine the age of peak performance among experts and to ascertain whether this age varies with level of expertise. Longitudinal designs can also be used to disentangle cohort and developmental changes associated with age and to investigate whether these effects are moderated by expertise. Few of these latter studies exist.

Expertise and Age in Sport and Games

Age-related changes in perceptual-motor and cognitive abilities (especially speed of processing) may limit high levels of performance among older experts in sport domains compared to other domains. A review of peak performance differences across different sports showed earlier peaks for more physically demanding sports such as swimming and sprinting than for less physically demanding sports such as golf (mid-20s vs. early 30s; Schultz & Curnow, 1988). Experience in sports with lower physical demands (golf, tennis) can reduce age-related differences on some perceptual-motor tasks. Coincident-timing tasks, especially tracking of accelerating targets, generally exhibit robust age declines. However, no significant age declines on such a task occurred for tennis players while declines did occur for nonplayers (Lobjois, Benguigui, & Bertsch, 2005). The authors argued that this pattern was due to a decrease in visual-motor delay in older players compared to nonplayers, which facilitated motor planning. There were similar delays for younger and older expert players, suggesting that high levels of practice maintained perceptual-motor skills. However, performance on domain-general tasks was not investigated, so it is possible that age-related benefits among expert players reflected more general factors, perhaps even effects of exercise on the elders' cognition (e.g., Colcombe et al., 2004).

Investigation of skilled performance in games (chess, bridge, Go) and in music provides further evidence that high levels of expertise can mitigate age differences under certain conditions. Master pianists do not exhibit age-related slowing on keyboard exercises, but they do on standard motor tasks (Krampe & Ericsson, 1996), consistent with the expertise literature demonstrating expertise benefits for domain-specific but not general tasks. In a study of movement planning among musicians of varying expertise, older amateur pianists simplified temporal sequencing in complex poly-rhythm tapping tasks to maintain global rate of performance, but older master pianists relied on parallel timing mechanisms (same vs. sequence of hands) to accommodate to the demands of changing to very rapid tempos (Krampe, Engbert, & Kliegl, 2002). These findings suggest that specific perceptual-motor strategies are maintained with age among high-level experts. Moreover, there was little evidence for age differences in these strategies among the experts, again consistent with a skill maintenance explanation for mitigation.

Skilled performance in chess also reflects perceptual and attentional strategies. Experts focus on relational versus item-specific properties of the most relevant pieces, with more information extracted per fixation (Charness et al., 2001). Moreover, recognition of chess moves is based on rapid retrieval from long-term memory of knowledge of configurations, helping to bypass working memory limitations (Ericsson & Kintsch, 1995). While high levels of skill did not reduce age-related slowing in time to detect a threat to the king in a recent study (Jastrzembski, Charness, & Vasyukova, 2006), age is often unrelated to effectiveness of search for chess moves among very expert players (Charness, 1981). More generally, high levels of expertise in chess, music, and related domains depend on deliberate practice, or investing large amounts of effort on individualized training activities designed to improve specific aspects of performance through repetition and successive refinement (Ericsson & Lehmann, 1996). Moreover, older experts appear to maintain superior performance through deliberate practice (Krampe & Ericsson, 1996).

In addition to person-based factors such as level of skill and deliberate practice, mitigation of age differences depends on task factors such as domain relevance. Domain-relevant tasks are organized in terms of domain constraints (Vicente & Wang, 1998) and thus are representative of the conditions under which experts usually perform (Ericsson, Patel, & Kintsch, 2000). Experts are likely to perform such tasks with little need for "overhead" operations in order to take advantage of domain knowledge, such as developing new representations or associating new responses to stimuli. Less domain-relevant tasks may penalize older experts because more cognitive resources are required to form new associations between aspects of the task and domain knowledge, or to map new responses to stimuli. For example, in contrast to the previously reviewed studies that investigated actual musical performance, tasks requiring recall of music material do not reveal mitigation (Halpern, Bartlett, & Dowling, 1995; Meinz & Salthouse, 1998; Meinz, 2000). Similarly, chess expertise is more likely to mitigate age differences for movement search tasks (a component of playing) than for recall tasks (Charness, 1981). Expertise in Go reduces age differences on reasoning or recognition but not on recall tasks (Masunaga & Horn, 2001). High levels of deliberate practice on domain-relevant tasks may help automatize perceptual-motor skills, and continued practice maintains these skills despite age-related declines in cognitive resources (Bosman & Charness, 1996). It is also possible that older experts increasingly rely on strategies such as anticipating task changes (Lobjois et al., 2005) or drawing inferences from information based on abstract problem representations (Ericsson & Lehman, 1996), which would suggest that compensatory strategies underlie mitigation.

In summary, studies of expertise in highly rule-governed domains such as sport and games suggest the importance of deliberate practice on perceptual-motor and attentional strategies for mitigating age differences in performance. More generally, as suggested by contextual approaches to cognition (Jenkins, 1979), mitigation appears to depend on characteristics of the person, the task, and the way performance is assessed.

Expertise and Aging Relations in Work-Related Domains

We next review work-related task domains that, similar to games, depend heavily on perceptual-motor skills. We then consider work domains in which performance also depends on a variety of cognitive skills such as planning and task management. Such domains may offer a wider range of paths to success for older experts.

Expertise tends to mitigate age differences on work-related tasks that are representative of expert performance. Age differences in one study occurred for novice, but not experienced, participants on an industrial drilling task (Murrell, 1970), although general cognitive abilities were not measured in this study so it is possible the absence of age effects among the experts reflected selection effects. More definitive evidence comes from Salthouse's (1984) classic study of transcription typing, in which performance was unrelated to age for typists with high levels of experience. The same participants showed typical age-related slowing on standard manual reaction time measures, suggesting that older experts were not selected for domain-general abilities. Information-processing limits that are typical of serial reaction time tasks appeared to be offset because typists could "look ahead" while executing keystrokes. Older typists appeared to rely more than younger typists on the preview strategy to offset slower motor processes, which suggested a compensatory strategy (also see Bosman, 1993). Similarly, among medical technicians, age-related declines were reduced on a domain-relevant visual search task (search for bacterial targets in a stain) but not on a domain-general visual search task (Clancy & Hoyer, 1994). Mitigation was more likely to occur among medical technicians when target identification was supported by congruent contextual cues (Hoyer & Ingolfsdottir, 2003), providing further evidence that expertise-based mitigation depends on the domain relevance of the task or the extent to which the task reflects domain constraints. These visual search studies did not identify the strategies underlying mitigation.

As we saw with expertise in chess and other games, mitigation is less likely for less domain-relevant work tasks, for example when performance in work domains requiring spatial ability (e.g., architecture) is measured by standard spatial ability tests (e.g., visualization, mental rotation). Age differences are comparable for samples varying in experience on tasks requiring these spatial abilities, either when experience is measured by self-rating (Salthouse, 1991) or when novices are compared to professionals whose practice requires these abilities (Salthouse et al., 1990 for architects; Lindenberger, Kleigl, & Baltes, 1992 for graphic designers).

Many work-related domains involve decision making under uncertainty, task management, problem solving, and other dimensions of "substantive complexity" (Schooler, Mulatu, & Oates, 1999). Moreover, collaboration is often critical because many work tasks are accomplished by teams rather than individuals. These domains may afford a variety of paths to maintaining competence among older experts, especially because performance in these domains depends more on consistent levels of effort than the peak performance that is often required to excel in sport and games (see Ackerman, 1994 for a related distinction between maximal and typical performance). This review focuses on research in aviation and financial domains.

Because many work domains are closely related to public safety, financial well-being, and other socially important outcomes, there is interest in whether these outcomes are compromised among older expert workers. Similar to the finding that age is often unrelated to worker performance (e.g., Salthouse & Maurer, 1996), there is little evidence that age is associated with the incidence of accidents among experienced pilots (Li et al., 2003, 2006) and air traffic control specialists (Broach & Schroeder, 2006). However, age-related conclusions from these studies are limited by narrow age ranges (in part due to age-based retirement rules) and by the ability to distinguish effects of age, experience, and exposure to risk (Tsang, 2003). Global measures such as accident rates may also obscure age-related differences in error, efficiency, or other aspects of performance. We next review more focused studies that examine age–expertise relationships associated with cognitive components and strategies of work-related tasks.

Expertise mitigates age differences in the ability to allocate attention to multiple tasks, a component of task management essential to safe performance in piloting and other complex work domains (Adams, Tenney, & Pew, 1995). Pilot expertise reduces age differences in performing concurrent tasks such as manual tracking and short-term memory search, presumably because time-sharing mechanisms such as flexibly allocating attention in response to shifting priorities are supported by experience in performing concurrent piloting tasks (Tsang & Shaner, 1998; also see Lassiter et al., 1997). More generally, training in time sharing (e.g., variable-priority training) reduces age differences in the performance of concurrent tasks (Kramer et al., 1999).

Expertise reduced age differences on a laboratory pilot–controller communication task in which participants listened to and read back complex air traffic control (ATC) messages (a common pilot communication procedure), in part because pilots relied on domain knowledge to integrate message and contextual information to create a dynamic mental model of the flight situation (Morrow et al., 1994). This finding is consistent with research showing that older adults differentially benefit when they can draw on domain knowledge to draw inferences leading to situation models (e.g., Miller et al., 2004).

Because accurate mental models of flight situations underlie effective pilot decision making (Orasanu & Fischer, 1997), expertise may mitigate age differences in decision making as well as communication. Participants in one study read flight scenarios at their own pace and then identified problems in the scenarios and appropriate responses to these problems (Morrow et al., 2008). Older airline pilots were as likely as their younger counterparts to identify solutions to problems, while age differences occurred for less experienced pilots. Younger and older experts were also more likely than novices to slow down when reading problem-relevant information, consistent with studies showing that experts focus on relevant cues.

As mentioned at the outset of the chapter, expertise is rooted as much in external as in internal strategies (Hutchins, 1995; Kirlik, 1995). Pilots are adept at interacting with their environment to reduce task demands on vulnerable cognitive resources such as working memory; for example, they use external aids such as note taking when communicating with ATC. Age differences in read-back accuracy were eliminated for pilots but not for nonpilots when participants could take notes while listening to the ATC messages, in part because older and younger pilots took more accurate and elaborate notes (Morrow et al., 2003; also see Morrow et al., 2008). Such findings suggest that mitigation is more likely when pilots take advantage of domain-relevant environmental support to reduce the need for self-initiated cognitive processing that declines with age (Craik & Jennings, 1992). More generally, older adults in a variety of work domains maintain performance over time by developing expertise in environmental supports, from external aids to a web of collaborative relationships with colleagues (Park, 1994).

Opportunity to draw upon both external and internal expert strategies may be reduced when performance is assessed in impoverished laboratory environments, with performance measures that do not tap knowledge-based representations or that require participants to invest additional cognitive resources to map these representations onto task requirements. For example, mitigation is not observed in studies testing recall of domain-relevant text in aviation (Morrow, Leirer, & Altieri, 1992) as well as other domains (Hambrick & Engle, 2002). Task complexity and method of assessment influence when expertise mitigates age differences. Mitigation is less likely on pilot–controller communication tasks involving complex procedures and materials that increase demands on pilots' working memory (Morrow et al., 2005 vs. Morrow et al., 1994).

Relationships between pilot age and expertise have also been investigated in the context of realistic simulated flight conditions that incorporate more domain-relevant constraints. Age differences in these studies among expert pilots are minimal for routine maneuvers such as maintaining level flight, perhaps because performance reflects highly practiced procedural skills (Taylor et al., 1994, 2005). Age differences are more apparent for less familiar tasks such as avoiding encroaching aircraft, or for ATC communication tasks that place heavy demands on pilots' working memory, especially when pilots do not have recourse to external aids (as in the laboratory studies mentioned earlier).

Few studies have investigated age–expertise relationships over time, using a longitudinal research design that would help disentangle cohort and developmental effects on performance associated with advancing age, and the ways in which experience moderates these effects. Taylor and colleagues (2007) used a longitudinal design to investigate age and expertise effects on performance in a light aircraft flight simulator for a sample of pilots age 40 to 69 years at study entry. Over a three-year testing period, more expert pilots (more advanced flight ratings) performed better at baseline and were less likely to decline over the testing period. Older pilots performed less well than younger pilots at baseline, with age differences most apparent on demanding ATC communication tasks. However, the extent of age-related difference was not reduced by expertise, although it was difficult to detect mitigation effects because there were relatively few pilots at the older and more experienced end of the sample distribution. Surprisingly, older pilots were less likely to decline over time than younger pilots were, although it is unclear why this was the case (e.g., regression to the mean; age-related benefits of repeated testing). Nonetheless, the study provides provocative findings regarding change in performance over time for pilots of varying age and skill level.

Expertise mitigates age differences for ATC specialists as well as pilots. Air traffic control requires perceptual and attention skills such as detecting and resolving conflicts between aircraft represented on radar displays, as well as more complex task management and planning skills. Expertise mitigation in one study was most likely to occur for more realistic tasks that required complex task management skills such as issuing instructions to control aircraft, even though controllers as well as noncontrollers experienced typical age-related declines on measures of the cognitive abilities required for the ATC tasks (Nunes, 2006). Older controllers had operational error rates similar to those of the younger controllers but issued fewer commands to the controlled aircraft, suggesting more efficient control as a potential compensatory strategy. Air traffic control specialists routinely perform these complex control tasks on a daily basis, and this high level of experience may be more likely to engender compensatory strategies than on pilots' performance of similarly complex (but less frequently performed) tasks. However, similar strategies and benefits might occur for complex tasks routinely performed by airline pilot crews, although researchers have yet to investigate potential age-related benefits of collaboration among airline pilots.

To sum up, investigations of age and expertise in the aviation domain suggest that mitigation occurs not only because older experts with high levels of current experience maintain procedural knowledge (similar to findings from studies of chess and related domains), but also because they develop strategies such as the use of external aids that support planning. More studies are needed that investigate how older and younger aviators perform complex tasks under controlled but realistic conditions in order to identify age differences in strategies related to decision making, task management, and situation awareness (Hardy & Parasuraman, 1997).

Studies of expertise in the financial domain also suggest that older adults maintain high levels of competence through a variety of strategies. Financial expertise is increasingly important because adults spend more and more years of their life in retirement, often depending on financial investments. There is mixed evidence as to whether older adults' financial competence is supported by knowledge and experience in the financial domain. Older adults who invest appear to know more than younger adults about investment principles such as diversifying portfolios, but these older investors are also less skilled at maintaining diverse portfolios by selecting stocks, perhaps because of age-related losses in cognitive resources that would support these skills (Korniotis & Kumar, 2005). If this finding is correct, experience and training in financial decision making might offset these cognitive declines. Hershey, Jacobs-Lawson, and Walsh (2003) found that 8 hr of training in financial decision making eliminated age differences in solving financial investment problems related to retirement investing, while age differences occurred among untrained participants. Analysis of problem-solving strategies showed that trained individuals, regardless of age, used similar efficient information search strategies that reflected the development of abstract problem representations.

These studies are somewhat limited by laboratory assessment of the benefits of financial expertise and training, with few performance measures. Investigating how financial experts accomplish workplace goals may reveal a broader range of expert strategies that mitigate age-related declines in cognitive processes and that support competence. A study of bank managers varying in age and expertise (measured by outcomes such as salary and promotions, as well as supervisor ratings) showed that, for the most expert participants, age was unrelated to performance on a measure of management knowledge, while age-related declines occurred on a fluid mental ability measure regardless of level of expertise. Moreover, the management knowledge measure predicted successful management outcomes only for the more expert participants (Colonia-Willner, 1998). This study suggests the importance of knowledge garnered from experience for supporting high levels of competence on the job; and because the knowledge measure tapped collaborative strategies, it also suggests the importance of collaboration for mitigating age differences on complex work tasks.

Conclusions

The studies reviewed in this chapter provide reason to be optimistic about the benefits of knowledge and skill for supporting high levels of performance on daily tasks in the face of age-related changes in the cognitive abilities necessary to perform those tasks. At the same time, the studies suggest caution because the extent of these benefits is circumscribed by biologically based sensory and cognitive declines associated with aging. Expertise can reduce age differences on a variety of complex tasks, but a confluence of factors related to the person (e.g., skill level, amount of deliberate practice), the task (e.g., domain relevance, difficulty), and the method of assessment (e.g., recall or reasoning) influences the extent of mitigation. Moreover, the paths to mitigation may vary with the domain of expertise. For domains that are heavily circumscribed by rules and in which perceptual-motor and attentional skills play a critical role (sport, games, work tasks such as typing), mitigation is most likely to be seen when high levels of deliberate practice help maintain these skills. For domains requiring a variety of complex cognitive skills, there may be more diverse paths to mitigation. For example, in aviation, some components of piloting are highly automatized (maintaining level flight), while other more cognitively demanding components (pilot communication and decision making) may be supported by skilled use of external aids and other task management strategies. Managerial work positions often require sophisticated collaborative strategies, and successful older managers maintain high levels of competence by developing collaborative expertise, which may be more tacit knowledge gained on the job than directly taught (Colonia-Willner, 1998). Older adults may be especially adept at acquiring this knowledge because of age-related gains in knowledge and wisdom linked to interpersonal relationships (Baltes & Staudinger, 1993; Hess et al., 2005).

Less positively, the expertise literature suggests that the mitigating effects of expertise are circumscribed in at least two ways. First, there is little evidence that general cognitive abilities are spared or remediated by experience on specific tasks that require these abilities, although most studies are not designed to directly test this issue because expert and nonexpert samples are selected with the hope of *not* finding differences on general cognitive measures (which would raise issues of selection effects). Second, a theme of this chapter has been that expertise mitigates age differences for domain-relevant tasks, with fewer age-related benefits for domain-general tasks (e.g., Clancy & Hoyer, 1994) or even for tasks with domain-relevant materials that are usually not performed by experts (Morrow et al., 1994).

The finding that the scope of mitigation is limited to domain-relevant conditions echoes evidence that the benefits of expertise (e.g., Ericsson & Lehmann, 1996) and cognitive training (Ball et al., 2002) are narrowly circumscribed. All of this work contrasts with studies of physical, intellectual, and social engagement, which tend to show broader benefits, in that experience on multifaceted complex tasks is associated with maintaining and sometimes improving component cognitive abilities (for review see Stine-Morrow et al., in press). This contrast may relate to the fact that experts typically deploy skills in relatively circumscribed conditions with a predictable range of demands, in which strategies and resources are used to obtain specific goals rather than to build capacities. To the extent that learning (Bjork, 1999) or complex expertise domains (e.g., work, Schooler et al., 1999) engender broad approaches to meeting the complex demands of diverse goals, broader benefits of expertise for older adults' cognition may occur.

CHAPTER 5

Exercise Effects on Learning and Neural Systems

Brenda J. Anderson, PhD
*Department of Psychology and the Program in Neuroscience,
SUNY Stony Brook*

Daniel P. McCloskey
Department of Psychology, City University of New York, Staten Island

Nefta A. Mitchell
Department of Psychology, SUNY Stony Brook

Despina A. Tata
Department of Psychology, Aristotle University of Thessaloniki

The present chapter reviews research on exercise effects on the brain with the goal of addressing whether these effects on cognition are a consequence of selective effects of exercise on specific neural systems or an indirect consequence of general hormonal and vascular responses to exercise. Exercise could have widespread effects on hormonal, immune, and cardiovascular systems that in turn influence the brain. Here we explore how exercise influences four brain areas. Three areas are related to movement; and the fourth area, the hippocampus, is more closely associated with cognitive functions. Within motor systems, exercise has been shown to affect neuronal and metabolic variables. In the hippocampus, exercise has been shown to affect the proliferation and survival of new neurons and growth factor expression, but not metabolic capacity. We explore the possibility that these effects are mediators of exercise effects on cognition. Together the data suggest that exercise selectively influences brain areas and therefore that selective effects could directly mediate cognitive improvement.

The possibility that physical activity could influence the brain is not new to the field of neuroscience. In 1893, Tanzi wrote, "[A] nerve impulse that passes more frequently through a neural connection will provoke hypernutrition of the overexcited pathways . . . there will follow a hypertrophy. . . ."

Research support has been provided by MH57845 and MH62075. Nefta Mitchell is supported by a W. Burghardt Turner Fellowship. We would like to thank Janette Ponticello and Doreen Olvet for help with the manuscript.

Cajal in 1911 (Ramon Y Cajal,w et al.,1988) agreed with Tanzi (1893), but added that such a mechanism cannot explain the skills developed by experts and their ability to develop new motor sequences. Whereas Tanzi focused on change at existing synapses, Cajal suggested "the establishment of other new pathways, by means of branching and progressive growth. . . ." Although Tanzi and Cajal were both considering brain alterations related specifically to movement-related areas of the brain, the current volume considers an additional question. Does exercise influence cognitive as well as motor systems, and if so, how?

To address how exercise might influence cognition, we need to study the brain in addition to learning. Thus animal models, which allow invasive methods, are reviewed in this chapter. Evidence for the ability of exercise to influence cognition in animals is also reviewed. Then exercise-induced brain alterations in both motor and nonmotor areas are discussed. Since exercise influences many biological systems (cardiovascular, immune, and neural systems), this review addresses whether exercise-induced changes in the brain are specific to brain regions or are general and therefore more likely to be a result of vascular or hormonal responses to exercise. In addition, we review research specifically dealing with signaling systems that may mediate exercise-induced improvements in cognition.

Animal Models of Exercise

Models of aerobic exercise in rodents take two forms, voluntary exercise in running wheels attached to the home cage and forced walking or running on a treadmill. Forced swimming, used less often, is employed both to force exercise and as a stressor. Therefore, the interpretation of results from studies that used forced swimming is not straightforward, and these studies are excluded from this review. For wheel running and treadmill training there is no standard paradigm. In the voluntary exercise condition, rats, mice, and gerbils usually have access to a running wheel 24 hr per day (Black et al., 1990; Neeper et al., 1996; McCloskey et al., 2001), seven days a week, although some investigators give access to running wheels for only 3 hr a day (Lambert et al., 2005). The duration of the exercise treatment condition can be short (e.g., two days) (Neeper et al., 1996) or long (e.g., six months) (McCloskey et al., 2001). When rats are forced to run on a treadmill, daily run times are usually 1 hr for five to seven days a week. Running speeds can vary from a rapid walk (10 m/min) (Isaacs et al., 1992) to running (27 m/min) (Gilliam et al., 1984). The faster speeds are often used to produce running speeds that require 70% to 90% of the maximum oxygen consumption ($\dot{V}O_2$max) (Spirduso and Farrar, 1981; Gilliam et al., 1984). The duration of treadmill treatments can range from one month (Isaacs et al., 1992) to six months (MacRae et al., 1987b).

For animals, running on a treadmill, like swimming, is forced rather than voluntary exercise. As a result, it may be stressful. Typically two strategies are employed to reduce the stress. First, all animals for the study are placed on a treadmill and forced to run before the study is begun. The animals that refuse to run are excluded from the study, and the remaining animals are divided into the running and control conditions (Spirduso and Farrar, 1981). A second strategy involves slowly increasing the speed and duration of running over several weeks until the animals in the exercise condition are trained to run the desired speed and duration (Isaacs et al., 1992). In studies using high speeds of running, shock can be used to motivate running. Unfortunately, investigators do not always report the number of shocks administered, so it is unclear how shock influences the nature of the treatment. The concerns over the possibility of psychological stress in the forced-exercise condition explain the preference for voluntary exercise in the recent literature in this field.

Similar to the studies of exercise in humans, studies of exercise in animals can include measurements of one or two variables that can be used to confirm improvements in fitness. Ideally, an investigator would show that the maximum oxygen consumption has increased after training (e.g., Spirduso and Farrar, 1981), but the equipment needed for these measures is expensive. Some investigators have measured the capacity for energy production in muscles by measuring metabolic enzymes (e.g., cytochrome oxidase activity) (Gilliam et al., 1984). Unfortunately, these latter measures are not available to all labs, and may not be compatible with specialized fixation methods required for the preservation of brain tissue. Fortunately, muscle, adrenal gland, and heart weight provide a simple third alternative for the measure of fitness (Isaacs et al., 1992). These measures are economical and compatible with most experimental methods. With the use of running wheels, the amount of running in the wheel is not under the control of the experimenter, and therefore evidence of conditioning is even more important in these studies than in studies utilizing treadmill training.

Can Exercise Influence Rodent Cognition?

It is a challenge to determine whether or not exercise affects cognition in rodents. The rodent behavior closest to requiring "cognition" is spatial learning and memory. Spatial learning is dependent upon the hippocampus, a structure that is believed to be involved in declarative forms of memory in humans and to associate items that are discontiguous over space and time in rodents (Wallenstein et al., 1998).

Early studies addressing the relationship between physical activity and cognitive ability tested whether "smarter" animals were more active. Using sheep, Lidell (1925) failed to find a correlation between number of steps taken per day by sheep and their ability to exit a maze. Likewise, Shirley (1928) failed to find evidence in rats that performance in a Lashley-type maze could predict activity in a rotating cage during the five days after maze testing. Runquist and Heron (1935) compared maze performance and activity in 17th-generation rats bred for high and low activity. Those animals that had higher activity rates in running wheels during the two weeks preceding maze testing made fewer errors. In a more recent study, mice selected for high running rates (generations 25 and 27) had learning curves similar to those of control mice (Rhodes et al., 2003). In the latter study, unlike that of Runquist and Heron (1935), neither group was given an opportunity to run, so the results are easier to interpret. Overall, the data suggest that there is no relationship between a predisposition to run and learning ability.

To experimentally examine whether exercise could improve cognition, many investigators have tested whether exercise can influence spatial memory. Spatial memory can take two forms, working memory and reference memory. Working memory is a transient form of memory usually tested within trials or across two trials within a day. Reference memory is a longer-lasting form of memory that is usually tested over days. In one form of testing, the Morris water maze, rats must learn the position of an escape platform submerged in a pool of water. Rats naturally use visual spatial cues outside of the maze to form a cognitive map that is utilized to find the location of the platform. The place-learning set version is used to test spatial working memory. In this version, rats learn a new goal position on the first trial of each pair of trials. On the second trial, memory for the position on trial 1 is tested. Fordyce and Farrar (1991b) found that forced treadmill training at a speed of 20 m/min (0% grade) for 60 min for 14 weeks (five days per week) improved the ability of rats to find the submerged platform by as much as 2- to 12-fold relative to the performance of sedentary rats. Similar results have been reported for mice that were forced to run in a treadmill (12 m/min, 0% grade, 60 min per day for five days per week) for eight weeks (Fordyce and Wehner, 1993). In both studies the groups did not differ in their swim speed. Therefore, differences in physical fitness do not appear to account for the improved performance. In another study, spatial working memory was improved in mice when access was provided to running wheels for only 3 hr a day over a period of three to six weeks (Lambert et al., 2005).

The swim speed data suggest that differences in physical fitness could not account for the group differences in spatial working memory. However, other effects of exercise could also potentially confound the results. For example, exercise is a physical stress hypothesized to enhance an organism's response to other stressors (Sothmann et al., 1996), and forced swimming is considered a stressor. Differences in the response to forced swimming, which would elevate glucocorticoids—hormones that can affect memory—could account for differences in task performance.

To avoid the potential confound from differences in the response to stress, an appetitive spatial learning task has also been used to test for exercise-related improvements in spatial learning. In this task, rats with restricted access to water obtain drops of water at the end of each of eight arms. The rats naturally learn to remember which arms they have entered during a single trial in order to retrieve the water efficiently. Consequently, repeat entries into arms where drops have already been consumed are considered errors. Unlike the water maze, rats in this task are not motivated by efforts to remove an aversive stimulus, and therefore the rats are not under time pressure. Thus differences in physical ability are less likely to influence performance and attention in the eight-arm maze than in the water maze. In this paradigm, female rats that voluntarily ran in wheels attached to their home cage for seven weeks had greater heart weights and acquired criterion-level performance on the eight-arm maze in significantly fewer days than littermate controls (Anderson et al., 2000b). The two groups did not differ in the amount of time it took to traverse each arm of the maze. To test whether the additional spatial experience in the home cage influences spatial processing, a follow-up study included one group of rats with access to locked wheels attached to the home cage. In this study, rats with locked wheels required the same number of trials to reach criterion as control rats and significantly more trials than exercise rats (unpublished observations; see figure 5.1). In both studies, once rats reached criterion performance, the performance of the two groups no longer differed. The data suggest that exercise gave the voluntary running group an early but not a late advantage. A concern was that the exercise group might be more motivated to obtain the water droplets, so the water restriction regimen

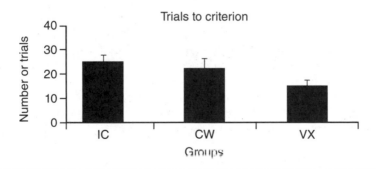

Figure 5.1 Exercise (VX) rats required fewer trials to reach criterion performance in the eight-arm radial maze than rats in the control condition (IC) or rats with access to locked wheels (CW). Criterion performance was defined as seven correct arm entries out of the first eight trials on four of five consecutive days.

was changed over studies in an effort to control for the possibility of differential deprivation. The similarity in performance across groups on trials after criterion was reached suggests that the rats from the two groups were equally motivated to perform the task. The learning data from the radial maze are consistent with findings from the Morris water maze.

Exercise has also been shown to influence reference memory. In one test of this form of memory, subjects have to find the same goal position in trials that occur across days in the Morris water maze. Fordyce and Wehner (1993) using treadmill training, and later van Praag using voluntary exercise (van Praag et al., 1999a, 1999b), found that the rodents that exercised had fewer spatial reference memory errors. Swim speed did not differ between the two groups in either study. These findings have been replicated numerous times (Rhodes et al., 2003; Adlard et al., 2004; Griesbach et al., 2004; Vaynman et al., 2004). When running wheels were used in the previous studies, rodents had daily access for 24 hr. However, when wheel access was limited to 3 hr a day for a three- to six-week period, exercise improved working but not reference memory (Lambert et al., 2005). It is unclear whether more exercise is necessary to enhance reference memory than working memory. Both forms of spatial learning are believed to be dependent, in part, on the hippocampus. Thus if exercise affects spatial learning, it is likely to affect the hippocampus.

One study failed to report an effect of exercise on spatial memory. Using young (6 months old) and old rats (27 months old), Barnes and colleagues (1991) tested the influence of exercise on spatial learning ability. Rats in the exercise condition were trained to run in a treadmill for 1 hr per day for five days per week over 10 weeks. Rats ran at a speed equal to 75% of their maximal oxygen consumption, a regimen that increased the heart-to-body weight ratio. After training, the animals were able to run faster at maximal capacity than prior to exercise training. The rats were tested on a Barnes maze, which is a circular platform with holes around the periphery. A darkened goal box is placed under one hole of the maze, and as in the standard version of the Morris water maze, rats are required to find this single goal position using reference memory. Unlike the water maze, the Barnes maze uses only mildly aversive stimuli, a well-lit room and a white platform, to entice the animal into a dark, safe goal box. In this study, the investigators used the same goal location for the first 13 trials and then changed the goal position for trials 14 through 17. They reported only the number of errors averaged over days 11 through 13 and on trial 17—trials that reflect well-learned responses. The authors found no effect of exercise in this study. These results are in agreement with the failure to find effects of exercise after animals achieved criterion-level performance in the eight-arm radial maze study (Anderson et al., 2000b). It would be interesting to know whether exercise can influence the number of trials required to reach criterion performance in the Barnes maze, because the task tests spatial memory without the need for physical exertion or deprivation.

A recent study of mice selected to run in wheels yielded surprising results. High runners were selectively bred for 25 to 27 generations (Rhodes et al., 2003). Female mice were given wheels from postnatal days 29 through 69. During the last six days they were trained in the Morris water maze. Among control mice, runners performed better than nonrunners as previously demonstrated. However, among mice selected for high running rates, runners were not statistically different from nonrunners and had a tendency to perform less well. Whereas the failure to find a consistent link between running and learning calls into question a causal relationship, it is also possible that the selectively bred mice are no longer representative of the larger population of mice.

Other investigators have tested exercise effects on behaviors that are far less likely to reflect exercise influences on the body and cardiovascular system. For example, testing conditioned reflexes provides the opportunity to study acute responses that require less energy than swimming or walking in a maze. In a well-designed study, auditory and contextual fear conditioning were measured in control rats and rats that voluntarily exercised in running wheels for 30 days (Baruch et al., 2004). The two groups exhibited similar freezing rates during paired presentations of an auditory stimulus and shock. After training, the two groups had similar freezing responses to the auditory stimulus, but exercise rats had greater freezing rates to the context. This latter form of conditioning, contextual fear conditioning, is dependent upon the hippocampus. Taken together, the findings suggest that the exercise rats had no greater sensitivity to shock or auditory stimulus but were better able to associate a context with fear. It is interesting to note that not all forms of learning were enhanced by exercise, only the form dependent upon the hippocampus. Van Hoomissen and colleagues (2004) also tested exercise effects on contextual fear conditioning. In this study, rats with access to exercise wheels also froze more in a context associated with shock, although only in the first 3 min. Together, both studies support the finding that exercising rats freeze more to a context associated with fear, a form of conditioning, like spatial learning, that is dependent upon the hippocampus.

Although Baruch and colleagues (2004) found that exercise does not influence the percent of responses to stimuli, Spirduso and Farrar's (1981) data suggest that exercise may influence the speed of the response. To test whether exercise improves reactive avoidance, Spirduso and Farrar (1981) had rats run up to 30 m per minute for 60 min a day over a period of eight weeks. The effectiveness of the training protocol is supported by their finding that oxygen utilization in muscle increased in both the young and old trained rats relative to controls. Treadmill training reduced both the latency to release a lever *after* shock and the latency to release a lever *to avoid* shock (Spirduso and Farrar, 1981).

Behavior changes with age, and exercise may be able to attenuate such age-related changes. The percent of correct avoidance responses on a reactive avoidance task was reduced by age in control but not in exercising rats (Spirduso and Farrar, 1981). Spontaneous activity decreased after the age of 10 months in rats and continued to decline. Treadmill training from 5 to 23 months attenuated the age-related declines in spontaneous activity (Skalicky et al., 1996). Another study showed that frequent lower-intensity exercise was more effective than intermittent high-intensity exercise at reducing the age-related declines (Skalicky and Viidik, 1999).

In summary, studies in animals indicate that exercise can influence performance on learning and memory tasks, reactive avoidance speed, and spontaneous activity. It is particularly difficult to control for potential differences in motivation, the response to stress, and changes in attention and vigilance. Until all of these are ruled out, it is possible to question whether exercise influenced learning per se or factors that indirectly influence learning. Consequently, the most convincing evidence that exercise improves learning comes from reports showing that exercise influences contextual fear conditioning. If the biological mechanism for learning to fear a context is the same as the mechanism used for more complex learned responses (e.g., spatial learning), as we assume it is, then it is safer to conclude that spatial learning improvements seen after exercise are indeed improvements in learning. Next, we will consider what types of plasticity are seen in brain regions associated with movement and spatial learning, and whether there are forms of plasticity that could serve as mediators of exercise-related improvements in learning.

Brain Structures Active During Exercise and Influenced by Exercise

Specific movements are controlled by motor regions of the brain, including the cerebellum, striatum, and motor cortex. In this chapter, we focus on exercise effects in the three motor regions. Spatial learning is dependent upon the hippocampus. This structure has neural activity related to movement, but is associated more closely with complex behavioral tasks such as spatial learning and memory.

It is important to consider that exercise may influence the brain not just through neuronal activity selectively associated with movement planning and proprioceptive feedback, but also through activation and adaptation in other systems. Activation of the sympathetic nervous system and endocrine systems, which increases blood flow, heart rate, and glucose availability, supports the energy demands of muscles. Exercise elevates adrenal hormones (Samorajski et al., 1987; Kjaer, 1998), which have bidirectional interactions with the brain and immune system. And exercise has been shown to affect the immune system (Fleshner et al., 2003): These effects include altered immune factor expression in the central nervous system (Campisi et al., 2003). Likewise, exercise effects on the cardiovascular system (Marsh and Coombes, 2005; Tousoulis et al., 2005) have implications for brain function when considered in light of the fact that the brain consumes at least 20% of total oxygen intake despite accounting for only 2% of body weight. Therefore, there are multiple pathways through which exercise effects on the body could influence the brain.

Improved cognition following habitual exercise could be mediated in one or more of the following ways: indirectly by hormonal, immune, or cardiovascular alterations; directly by neural activity related to movement production; or by somatosensory and proprioceptive feedback resulting from movement. If cognitive improvements from exercise are solely mediated by general cardiovascular and hormonal alterations, we would expect exercise-related brain plasticity to be broadly distributed. The following discussion of plasticity in brain structures that are active during exercise cites evidence to suggest that the changes are not broadly distributed, but instead can be localized to specific brain regions.

In order for exercise to influence cognition, it must have a long-lasting effect on the brain. Six forms of plasticity resulting from exercise have been studied; these include changes in (1) receptor density and neurotransmitter concentrations, (2) growth factor expression, (3) rates of cell division, (4) metabolism, (5) gene expression, and (6) cell survival after damaging events. Where possible, evidence for each form of plasticity is discussed for each of the brain regions included in this review. The forms of plasticity studied in each structure differ somewhat, in part because of the neurotransmitter systems in each structure and the topics of greatest interest at the time exercise-related influences in each structure were studied. Likewise, some structures have been studied more than others. The hippocampus has been the focus of many recent studies, not for a direct relationship to movement, but instead because of its relatively simple anatomical structure and its relationship to memory. As a result, it is important not to draw conclusions about missing data or to make assumptions about regional importance with regard to exercise based on the amount of data available.

Cerebellum

The cerebellum, a motor structure, controls posture and coordination. It also appears to integrate somatosensory and vestibular information to influence movement. Its activation during exercise is supported by findings that treadmill running in dogs increases cerebral blood flow in this region

(Gross et al., 1980). The cerebellum, like the visual cortex, undergoes structural alterations in response to enriched housing (Greenough, 1984). Because the enriched environment increases the opportunity for physical activity, researchers have tested whether exercise and skill learning separately influence the cerebellum. To differentiate the effects of learning and physical activity, Black and colleagues (1990) studied the effects of motor skill learning and exercise on the anatomical structure of the cerebellum. One group of rats traversed an obstacle course that required acquisition of new motor skills. To control for the amount of activity associated with the task, two exercise groups were used. In one, rats voluntarily ran in wheels attached to their home cages. In the other, rats were trained to walk rapidly in a treadmill for up to 1 hr per day. The strategy was to create very robust training on two different dimensions. If skill learning, but not exercise, influenced a variable such as synapse number, it would be difficult for skeptics to argue that the skill learning condition involved greater physical activity than the exercise conditions. Likewise, if exercise, a simple repetitive task with relatively little skill learning, influenced a variable, it would be difficult to argue that exercising rats could have learned more than the skill-learning rats. Structural alterations were investigated in the paramedian lobule (PML), which receives somatosensory input from forelimbs and hind limbs. In this region, the skill-learning group that traversed an obstacle course had a thicker molecular layer and a greater number of synapses per neuron in the molecular layer than the control, voluntary exercise, and forced-exercise groups (Black et al., 1990). Although the skill learning group spent only 15 mimutes a day learning new skills, they had more synapses than either exercise condition, including the condition with wheels available 24 hr a day. The selective association between learning and greater synapse numbers suggests that altering the number of synapses may be a mechanism for learning in the cerebellum.

Exercise, like skill learning, produced structural alterations; but the alterations took a different form than those observed after skill learning. Both the voluntary and forced-exercise conditions caused an increase in the density of capillaries in the PML, changes not seen after skill learning (Isaacs et al., 1992). These data suggest that the additional neural activity associated with running created a greater need for oxygen and glucose, which was met by an increase in capillary density.

Exercise is not expected to increase neuron number in adult rats, but it may spare neurons during aging. Male rats that ran on a horizontal treadmill at 20 m per minute from 5 to 23 months of age had 11% more Purkinje cells than sedentary controls (Larsen et al., 2000). No difference in the number of Purkinje cells was found between the exercising aged rats and young rats. These findings suggest that exercise prevents or delays cell loss in the cerebellum.

In summary, skill learning for a mere 15 min a day increases the number of synaptic connections in the cerebellar cortex; but exercise, even when distributed over 24 hr, has no such effect. Instead, exercise increases capillary density. Likewise, exercise can reduce age-related cell loss. No studies have tested whether skill learning can reduce age-related cell loss in this region.

Motor Cortex

Activation of the rat motor cortex during running has been demonstrated with metabolic measures. Treadmill running increases regional cerebral blood flow in the sensorimotor cortex in dogs (Gross et al., 1980). In rats, exercise has been shown to cause transient increases in local cerebral glucose utilization (Vissing et al., 1996).

Like the cerebellum, the rat motor cortex undergoes longer-term alterations in response to skill learning. The motor cortex undergoes synaptogenesis following motor learning (Kleim et al., 1996, 2004). Both exercise and skill learning increased motor cortical thickness (Anderson et al., 2000a). Although synapses were not counted in this study, the greater thickness found in the exercise group is consistent with the possibility that synapses were added, since synapse addition has been shown to correspond to increases in cortical thickness in a number of studies (Greenough, 1984; Black et al., 1990). Additional support for the hypothesis that increasing neuronal activity, without changing the pattern of activity, is sufficient to increase synapse numbers comes from studies in which electrical stimulation given over time was sufficient to increase synapse numbers and dendritic and axonal arborizations (Rutledge et al., 1974; Keller et al., 1992).

In addition to neuronal alterations, it is also possible that exercise influences vascular function in the motor cortex, as it did in the cerebellum. A number of studies have addressed whether exercise alters metabolic capacity in the motor cortex, with mixed results. In one study, exercise was matched to the forced-exercise condition that increased capillary density in the cerebellum (Isaacs et al., 1992). When rats were forced to walk on a treadmill for 1 hr a day at a rate of 11 m/min, with a 10 min break after the first 30 min, for 30 days, there was no increase in capillary density in hind limb representations within the motor cortex (unpublished observations). In contrast, however, Kleim and colleagues (2002) found greater capillary density in the forelimb representations of the motor cortex after rats were given access to running wheels for 30 days. Swain and colleagues (2003) used three indirect measures to test whether exercise increases capillary density in the forelimb areas of the motor cortex. Using two types of functional magnetic resonance imaging (fMRI), they found that signal changes in exercise rats, relative to control rats, were consistent with the possibility that voluntary exercise increased capillary perfusion or blood volume. As a third measure, they demonstrated higher antibody labeling for a protein expressed at high levels during blood vessel development. Taken together, the data suggest that voluntary exercise may increase capillary density, at least in forelimb regions of the motor cortex.

Increases in capillary density would be expected to increase blood volume, which should serve to increase the availability of oxygen and glucose. Taken in light of the known tight coupling between blood flow and metabolism, these findings lead to the hypothesis that there should be an increase in metabolic capacity. If so, the increase should be reflected as an increase in cytochrome oxidase activity, since the brain relies overwhelmingly on aerobic metabolism. The activity of the cytochrome oxidase enzyme is coupled to the production of adenosine triphosphate, the source of free energy in the brain. When spatial distribution is of interest, it is possible to indirectly measure cytochrome oxidase activity with a histochemical method. Using this method, McCloskey and colleagues (2001) showed that rats that had access to exercise wheels attached to their home cage for six months (from 5 to 11 months of age) had greater metabolic capacity in the motor cortex, but not in control regions of the brain.

In conclusion, like the cerebellum, the motor cortex is influenced by exercise and motor skill learning. In both structures, exercise alters variables related to metabolism. In the cerebellum, only skill learning increased the thickness of the outer layer of dendrites (Black et al., 1990); but in the motor cortex, exercise, like skill learning, was able to increase cortical thickness.

Striatum

The striatum consists of the caudate and putamen, two of the three nuclei that make up the basal ganglia (the caudate, putamen, and globus pallidus). The striatum processes input from the motor cortex and other cortical regions. It projects to motor cortical areas to influence the planning and the initiation of voluntary movements. One form of striatal dysfunction is seen in Parkinson's disease, in which diminished dopaminergic input leads to resting tremors, a slow shuffling gait, and difficulty initiating voluntary movement. Evidence that the striatum is active during movement has been demonstrated in both humans and rodents. In humans, regional cerebral blood flow in the striatum increases during voluntary movement (Roland et al., 1982). In rats, running on a treadmill at 85% of their maximal oxygen consumption increases local cerebral glucose uptake in the striatum (Vissing et al., 1996). Electrophysiological recording in this region during movement can provide details about the functional relationship between neuronal activity and the behavior produced. When rats walked on a treadmill, 61% of striatal neurons were continuously excited during

20 s of walking (Shi et al., 2004). A small population exhibited inhibition continuously during walking, while another population was active only during the initiation or termination of walking. The data suggest that the striatum and other regions within the basal ganglia are associated with execution of limb movements.

Exercise has been shown to affect striatal transmitter binding. Treadmill running (27 m/min at 0% grade for approximately 80% of the subject's maximum oxygen consumption for 1 hr per day over a period of six months) has been reported to increase the density of dopamine type 2 (D2) receptors in the striatum of adult rats (MacRae et al., 1987a). Treadmill running significantly increased the maximal oxygen consumption relative to that in control rats. In a similar study, D2 receptor binding was studied in aged rats (MacRae et al., 1987b). The rats were trained to run on a treadmill up to 20 m per min for 60 min per day for five days per week over 12 weeks. The metabolic capacity of the gastrocnemius-plantaris was increased by 27% in the old (21 months old) treadmill-trained group relative to the young (6 months old) untrained group. From 6 to 12 months, D2 receptor binding sites decreased in controls, but treadmill training reduced this age-related decrease. Exercise also influenced a dopamine metabolite, DOPAC. DOPAC increased with age, but treadmill training prevented this age-related effect. These studies indicate that forced exercise can alter receptor expression in adult animals, and that exercise can attenuate age-related changes in dopaminergic transmission.

The dopaminergic system is not the only neurotransmitter system in the striatum that is influenced by exercise. In young rats, treadmill training (25-30 m/min at 0% grade for 60 min each of six days per week for eight weeks) and voluntary exercise in running wheels elevated striatal concentrations of the inhibitory neurotransmitter GABA relative to values in nonrunning rats (Dishman et al., 1996). Activity wheel running reduced $GABA_A$ receptor binding, whereas the treadmill training did not (Dishman et al., 1996). These results are particularly interesting because activity wheel running, but not treadmill training, increased open-field activity. A relationship between open-field activity and $GABA_A$ density is supported by earlier findings that blocking $GABA_A$ receptors increases open-field locomotion (Plaznik et al., 1990). Thus, voluntary running effects on $GABA_A$ receptor density may account for the increased open-field activity.

No studies have yet tested whether exercise can alter the structure of striatal neurons, but studies testing the effects of the enriched environment suggest that neural structure in this region is modifiable. Enriched housing increases the number of spines, or sites of excitatory synaptic contact, on medium spiny neurons in the dorsolateral striatum (Comery et al., 1995). The neurons that have this morphological alteration are the neurons that are known to express dopamine receptors. Enrichment has also been shown to alter dopamine receptor binding. Two-year-old rats exposed to an enriched environment have a greater ratio of dopamine type 1 (D1) receptors to muscarinic acetylcholine (ACh) receptors, but no change in D2 receptors (Anderson et al., 2000a). Taken together with earlier studies showing that exercise can decrease age-related reductions in D2 receptor binding, this work suggests that amounts of physical activity exceeding the amount that occurs in the enriched environment may be required to elevate D2 receptor binding. Overall, the studies suggest that behavioral conditions can alter neuronal structure and receptor binding in the striatum.

If neuronal activity changes during exercise, it seems possible that the striatum may increase its capacity for metabolism in order to keep up with those periods of greater metabolic demand. Rats that exercised for six months had relatively greater metabolic capacity in the limb representations of the striatum (dorsolateral caudate) relative to control regions (McCloskey et al., 2001). Not only do these results suggest that neurons in the limb regions of the striatum in exercising rats have a greater metabolic capacity after six months of exercise than in control rats; they also indicate that exercise effects are restricted within the striatum to regions that are likely to have elevated neural activity during running.

Nerve cells store relatively little free energy, yet they have relatively high metabolic demand. As a result, the nervous system needs a constant supply of oxygen and glucose. Ischemia refers to a disruption in the blood supply, which can occur during obstructive and hemorrhagic stroke. If exercise alters the capacity for metabolism in limb representation of the striatum, then it may protect neurons during damaging events like ischemia, which challenge the capacity for metabolism. In support of that hypothesis, gerbils that ran for two weeks in a running wheel prior to a 15 min blockade of the carotid artery had only 50% cell loss in the limb representations of the striatum compared to 90% cell loss in control gerbils. All gerbils that ran prior to a 20 min blockade survived the trauma relative to only 21% of gerbils in the control group (Stummer et al., 1994). Similarly, treadmill training in rats prior to middle cerebral artery occlusion reduces infarct volume (Ding et al., 2005). There is some evidence consistent with the hypothesis that exercise confers its neuroprotective effects during reperfusion following ischemia (Li et al., 2004). However, more work is needed to determine which effects of exercise mediate this protection.

Exercise *following* damage may also reduce the damage and spare function of the striatum. Treadmill running for 30 min once a day for 10 days following hemorrhage within the striatum reduced infarct size compared to that seen in sedentary control rats (Lee et al., 2003). In another study, rats were required to run at 15 m/min for 15 min twice a day for 10 days or remain sedentary following dopamine depletion, a rodent model of Parkinson's disease. Treadmill running, relative to the sedentary condition, left dopaminergic transmission and limb use relatively spared (Tillerson et al., 2003). In a similar study, treadmill training for 40 min per day for 30 days following dopamine depletion attenuated the depletion, but produced no sparing of behavior (Poulton and Muir, 2005).

In summary, neural activity and glucose uptake increase in the striatum during exercise. Habitual exercise causes the striatum to undergo alterations in the density of some types of transmitter receptors, as well as alterations in the concentration of some transmitters and their metabolites. Likewise, exercise increases metabolic capacity in limb-related subregions. Exercise before or after a metabolic challenge or toxin exposure protects the striatum from cellular damage and in some cases spares limb use. After damage, exercise has been used to improve recovery in this region.

A number of these studies measured the whole striatum, leaving us to question whether the effects are selective to limb representations or distributed throughout the striatum. Selective distribution would support the possibility that neural activity directly related to movement production is driving plasticity, in contrast to the possibility that plasticity results from broader effects of exercise (e.g., hormonal or cardiovascular effects). Only one study (McCloskey et al., 2001) differentiated areas within the striatum that should be activated from those that should not be activated during exercise. The results of that study suggested that at least metabolic plasticity is restricted to areas with limb representations.

Hippocampus

Mediators of the effects of exercise on spatial learning, already reviewed, most likely occur in the hippocampus, because lesions of the hippocampus impair spatial learning. Cells in the hippocampus are activated by positions in space (Czurko et al., 1999) and appear to work together to form a cognitive map of space. As a result, the hippocampus is considered a structure that processes complex spatial information.

Although hippocampal function is associated with cognition, evidence suggests that movement information is integrated with other spatial information in the hippocampus to code the position in space. Jumping, running, and walking increase hippocampal electrophysiological activity (Bland and Vanderwolf, 1972; Vanderwolf, 1988). Likewise, indirect measures of neuronal activity suggest that neurons in this region are active during locomotion (De Bruin et al., 1990; Vissing et al., 1996). In addition to encoding the position in space, the rate of neuronal firing can encode the velocity of movement (Czurko et al., 1999). Treadmill running increases acetylcholine release in the hippocampus (Dudar et al., 1979). Conversely, when acetylcholine is injected into the hippocampus, rats begin to locomote (Mogenson and Nielsen, 1984); this finding suggests that the hippocampus could also play a role in the motivation for voluntary movement. It has been proposed that the hippocampus uses internal movement information as one method of coding the distance traveled, and therefore the position, in an environment (Wallace et al., 2002; Wallace and Whishaw, 2003).

Given that this structure is associated with cognition, it is of interest which forms of exercise-induced plasticity in the hippocampus can be associated with learning. It is important to remember, however, that forms of plasticity identified in the hippocampus following exercise have not received equal consideration for their potential role in learning enhancement. Likewise, close relationships between learning and some forms of plasticity do not necessarily exclude the possibility that other forms of plasticity are involved.

Chronic exercise, like acute exercise, influences hippocampal neurochemistry. Repeated running five days per week for 14 months causes choline uptake to decrease, whereas acute treadmill running elevates high-affinity choline uptake in the hippocampus (Fordyce and Farrar, 1991a). When chronic running was combined with spatial memory testing, high-affinity choline uptake was increased. Long-term training alone or combined with spatial memory testing increased acetylcholine receptor binding in the hippocampus (Fordyce and Farrar, 1991b). Acetylcholine receptor density also decreased with age, but the decrease was attenuated by chronic exercise in aging animals (Fordyce et al., 1991). The latter finding is consistent with the more general supposition that exercise can retard, and possibly even reverse, some forms of aging.

In addition to effects on transmitter systems, there is significant current interest in exercise effects on molecular signaling mechanisms that have been shown to protect the brain. Brain-derived neurotrophic factor (BDNF) and nerve growth factor (NGF) belong to the family of growth factors called neurotrophins. They support the growth of processes during development and have been shown to protect the brain from aging and damage. Free access to running wheels for two, four, or seven days rapidly increased the amount of mRNA for BDNF and NGF in the hippocampus and caudal cerebral cortex relative to that in control rats (Neeper et al., 1995, 1996). Smaller but still significant increases in BDNF occurred in the cerebellum and frontal cortex. Given the number of molecular systems within the hippocampus that could be influenced by exercise, it is of interest whether the upregulation of BDNF and NGF is part of a more general upregulation of gene expression. To address this question, it is possible to use new methods that measure the expression of hundreds of genes at once (Tong et al., 2001; Molteni et al., 2002). Using gene microarrays, Molteni and colleagues (2002) concluded that the most significant increases in gene expression occurred for BDNF, as well as genes for proteins that interact with BDNF. Whereas gene expression for BDNF was upregulated after 3, 7, and 28 days of exercise, gene expression for NGF was upregulated after only 3 days of exercise and not after 7 and 23 days of exercise. If the upregulation of mRNA is to alter function, then growth factor protein must be increased. Brain-derived neurotrophic factor protein concentrations appear to remain elevated for as long as rats have the opportunity to voluntarily run (Adlard et al., 2004).

Could neurotrophins mediate exercise-induced improvements in spatial memory? Nerve growth factor when infused into the hippocampus improves spatial learning (Fischer et al., 1987; Markowska et al., 1996; Pelleymounter et al., 1996; Jakubowska-Dogru and Gumusbas, 2005). However, in all of these studies, subjects were already deficient in learning (e.g., they were aged, or were young but impaired learners). Exercise-related elevations of NGF are short-lived relative to increases in BDNF. They last for only two days of exercise (Neeper et al., 1996), so NFG seems unlikely to influence learning after longer durations of exercise. Unlike NGF, BDNF protein expression appears to remain high as long as rats have the opportunity to run (Adlard et al., 2004).

In support of a BDNF role in learning enhancement, BDNF mRNA expression increases during training in a spatial learning task (Mizuno et al., 2000) and a hippocampal-dependent inhibitory avoidance task (Alonso et al., 2002b). In support of a causal role for BDNF in memory formation, BDNF infusion into the hippocampus facilitates long-term memory in a fear-motivated task (Alonso et al., 2002b). Furthermore, blocking BDNF protein production impairs spatial learning (Mizuno et al., 2000), and blocking BDNF binding to its receptors has been shown to impair a hippocampal-dependent inhibitory avoidance task (Alonso et al., 2002a, 2002b). In an elegant effort to test for a causal relationship between exercise-induced BDNF levels and enhanced learning, Vaynman and colleagues (2004) found that exercise-induced enhancement on a reference memory task in the Morris water maze was blocked when the action of BDNF was blocked. Altogether, there is compelling support for a BDNF role in exercise-induced improvements in learning.

In light of the strong support for a BDNF role in exercise-induced improvements in spatial memory, two studies yield surprising findings. One study showed that BDNF infusion did not improve learning in aged, cognitively impaired rats, whereas infusion of NGF did improve learning (Pelleymounter et al., 1996). It may be important to consider, however, that in the aged cognitively impaired rats, the deficits could result from dysfunction in the downstream effects of BDNF (e.g., too few receptors), so that memory dysfunction occurs despite elevations in BDNF. In another study, Rhodes and colleagues (2003) found that in mice selectively bred for high rates of wheel running there was no correspondence between spatial learning and BDNF levels. Running, whether in control mice or mice selectively bred for high rates of running, increased BDNF relative to values in both nonrunning groups (control and selectively bred mice); however, only the control runners had better spatial learning. It is possible that despite BDNF elevations, another learning system activated by running in selectively bred mice (e.g., striatum) biased the selectively bred mice toward using an ineffective strategy (White and McDonald, 2002). As long as these possibilities exist, the contradictory data fail to disprove a relationship between BDNF, exercise, and learning. Currently, despite contradictions in the literature, BDNF appears to be a strong candidate as one mediator of exercise-induced improvements in cognition, at least when the task requires the hippocampus.

Despite the increase in growth factor expression, no one has tested whether exercise might influence dendritic length or synapse numbers in the hippocampus. In one study, synaptophysin, which is a measure of vesicle number, was higher in mice with access to running wheels for 3 hr a day for six weeks (Lambert et al., 2005). These effects were restricted to the hippocampus; synaptophysin was not elevated in the cerebellum or striatum. Whereas these mice had fewer working memory errors in the Morris water maze, other conditions (e.g., enrichment) increased synaptophysin levels in the hippocampus without improving working memory. As a result, the correspondence between synaptophysin levels and working memory is not as close as would be expected if one were dependent upon the other.

The rate of cell division and the survival of the new neurons (i.e., neurogenesis) in the hippocampus can be increased by behavioral experiences, including enriched housing (Kempermann et al., 1997) and voluntary running (van Praag et al., 1999a). In the latter study, exercise was shown to enhance spatial learning, long-term potentiation of synapses, and neurogenesis in the same animals. If neurogenesis were a mechanism for learning, then exercise-induced increases in neurogenesis could explain how exercise influences learning. Unfortunately, the forms of memory enhanced by exercise are not forms of memory dependent upon neurogenesis. Only hippocampal-dependent trace eye-blink conditioning is as yet known to be dependent on new neurons (Shors et al., 2002). Thus a failure to see improved spatial memory despite exercise-enhanced neurogenesis (Rhodes et al., 2003), and the ability to see enrichment-enhanced contextual fear conditioning without enrichment-enhanced neurogenesis (Feng et al., 2001), are not surprising, because neither spatial memory nor contextual fear conditioning appears to be dependent upon neurogenesis (Shors et al., 2002). Taken together, these studies predict that exercise should speed the acquisition of trace eye-blink conditioning, but this has not been tested.

In the hippocampus, inhibited neurogenesis has been proposed to cause depression (Duman, 2004). This hypothesis is of interest in the context of exercise because levels of physical activity are inversely related to rates of depression (Martinsen et al., 1985; Goodwin, 2003). Exercise can be used to reduce symptoms of depression in adults and persons who are elderly (Blumenthal et al., 1999; Dimeo et al., 2001) and to reduce relapse rates

(Babyak et al., 2000). Since exercise has been shown to increase neu-rogenesis (van Praag et al., 1999a), it could reverse depression through this effect if depression were caused by inhibited neurogenesis. For that reason, it is worth reviewing the support for the hypothesis. Serotonin, hypothesized to be reduced in depression, increases neurogenesis, and depletion of serotonin reduces neurogenesis (Banasr et al., 2004). Stress, which often precedes the onset of depression, is a reliable inhibitor of neurogenesis (Tanapat et al., 2001). Antidepressants have been shown to block stress-induced inhibition of neurogenesis (Czeh et al., 2001; Malberg and Duman, 2003; Santarelli et al., 2003). In an effort to demonstrate that the effectiveness of an antidepressant is dependent upon its ability to increase neurogenesis, one study tested the effects of antidepressants when neurogenesis was inhibited. In this study, an antidepressant was used to successfully treat a rodent model of depression, but was ineffective when neurogenesis was blocked by irradiation (Santarelli et al., 2003). However, in another model of depression, the results were not as sup-portive of the hypothesis. Subjects were treated with inescapable shock, which was shown to reduce the rates of cell proliferation in the dentate gyrus. If reduced rates of neurogenesis cause depression, then all animals should have exhibited symptoms of depression. However, only a subset of animals exhibited the symptoms (Vollmayr et al., 2003). Until a causal relationship between inhibited neurogenesis and depression can be well established, it remains to be seen whether neurogenesis is the mechanism through which exercise reduces symptoms of depression.

The role that BDNF plays in depression has also been considered (Russo-Neustadt and Chen, 2005). Both exercise and antidepressants increase BDNF mRNA expression in the hippocampus (Russo-Neustadt et al., 2001). Combined therapy further increases BDNF mRNA levels above baseline values. Voluntary exercise can protect against stress-induced decreases in BDNF expression (Adlard and Cotman, 2004). It is not yet clear whether BDNF can cause a reduction in depressive symptoms, although there is a correlation between BDNF mRNA expression levels in one region of the hippocampus and rodent measures of depression (Russo-Neustadt et al., 2001).

Given the number of variables in the hippocampus that are modified by exercise, the increased neuronal activity during exercise, and the tight coupling between neural activity and metabolism, it seems possible that exercise might influence hippocampal metabolism. Molteni and colleagues (2002) showed marginal increases in gene expression for cytochrome oxidase subunits IV, V, VI, VIII, 4 of the 13 subunits, after seven days of exercise. In contrast, cytochrome oxidase subunits I, II, and III (3 of 13) were decreased in expression in male rats that exercised for three weeks (Tong et al., 2001). The 13 subunits must increase in a coordinated fash-ion to form a functional enzyme. To test whether the enzyme increased, we measured cytochrome oxidase reactivity. Whereas six months of wheel running increased metabolic capacity in the motor cortex and limb regions of the striatum, it did not change cytochrome oxidase reactivity in the hippocampus (McCloskey et al., 2001). Either there is a short, but not a prolonged, increase in metabolic capacity in the hippocampus after exercise, or changes in gene expression for some subunits do not represent changes in enzyme concentrations. We have also used treadmill training to test whether exercise increases hippocampal capillary density. Using parameters for treadmill training similar to the parameters that increased capillary density in the cerebellum (Isaacs et al., 1992), as well as sensitive measures, we failed to find changes in capillary density in the hippocampus after treadmill walking (unpublished observations). Although exercise alters the expression of genes related to metabolism, there is no evidence that the changes in gene expression reflect changes in the rate of metabolism in the hippocampus.

Exercise can protect the hippocampus from damaging events. Previously we mentioned that exercise spared neurons in the striatum from death caused by ischemia (Stummer et al., 1994). In that same study, 50% of neurons in the CA3 subregion of the hippocampus of exercising gerbils survived after 15 min of ischemia, whereas only 10% of neurons survived in the control gerbils. The sparing was restricted to CA3 and was not seen in CA1, a subregion of the hippocampus particularly vulnerable to ischemia.

Like the mechanism of damage in ischemia, seizures lead to cellular depolarization that triggers damaging events such as excess calcium influx. Long-term exercise leads to resistance to electrical stimulation capable of producing seizures (Arida et al., 1998). High-running rats that exercised for one month were less likely to develop status epilepticus after systemic injections of kainic acid, an excitotoxin, than nonrunners and low runners (unpublished observations). These studies suggest that exercise produces seizure resistance. Following seizures, animals that exercised had a lower frequency of subsequent spontaneous seizures, and the effect persisted over a period of at least 45 days after the cessation of exercise (Arida et al., 1999). Several studies have examined the number of hippocampal cells that survive exposure to an excitotoxin. Following injection of domoic acid, rats trained to run on a treadmill had less cell loss in the hippocampus (Carro et al., 2001). However, when kainic acid was injected directly into the hippocampus, exercise in female rats appeared to exacerbate cell loss (Ramsden et al., 2003). If the different outcomes are related to the differences in the route of drug administration, it is possible that somatic effects of exercise partially account for protection from seizures.

To summarize, the finding that exercise influences hippocampal-dependent spatial learning has led investigators to test the effects of exercise on many different variables in the hippocampus. Exercise effects include changes in transmitter receptors, growth factor expression, cell proliferation and survival, and neuron survival after ischemia, but not upregulation of metabolic capacity or increases in capillary density. Of the variables shown to change in response to exercise, BDNF elevations have the most experimental evidence supporting a role in exercise-related improvements in spatial working and reference memory.

Which Condition Is the Control Condition?

Many investigators question whether the control rather than exercise condition might be the treatment condition. After all, the laboratory cage does not emulate the typical life of feral rats, which are free to roam, face danger, forage for food, and cluster in groups, and many of these activities involve physical exertion. The control rodent instead lives in a large, clear tub with no opportunities for exercise or learning. Whether one chooses to interpret the findings described earlier as effects of exercise or deprivation from lack of exercise, the findings nonetheless suggest that the brain responds to the level of physical activity. Given that our current society tends to be much more sedentary than it should be, perhaps the laboratory conditions serve well in simulating activity levels in developed nations.

Implications for Aging

Whereas much of the work on exercise effects on nervous tissue has been performed in the brain, several studies suggest that exercise affects peripheral nerves during aging. Between 17 and 27 months of age in rats, the number of axonal fibers, axonal diameter, and fiber density decreased in peripheral nerves innervating the gastrocnemius muscle (Kanda and Hashizume, 1998). The age-related reductions were not seen in animals that swam for 30 min a day three times a week for 10 months. Wheel running in mice for 2 hr per day between 3 and 24 months of age did not alter the number of myelinated fibers in the posterior tibial nerve, a sensory nerve, but caused hypertrophy relative to values in sedentary aged mice (Samorajski and Rolsten, 1975). Thus, in aging, exercise may affect the quality of somatosensory input to be processed by the central nervous system.

In the central nervous system, there is evidence from a number of brain regions that exercise can attenuate or prevent age-related changes. Exercise was shown to attenuate or prevent age-related cell loss in the cerebellum, age-related changes in dopamine receptors and metabolites in the striatum, and age-related changes in acetylcholine receptor density in the hippocampus. Likewise, exercise was found to attenuate age-related declines in spontaneous activity. Relatively few studies have undertaken such long-term comparisons, but those that have done so suggest that generally exercise retards brain aging.

Recent magnetic resonance imaging volumetric measures of young and aging humans (Salat et al., 2004), along with histological measures of cortical thickness in monkeys, suggest that both the primary and association cortices thin with age (Peters et al., 1996, 2001). Cardiovascular fitness has been shown to relate to brain tissue loss in frontal, parietal, and temporal cortices (Colcombe et al., 2003). If exercise supports richer sensory and motor experiences, improved blood flow, and maintenance of neuronal integrity, then it may be that cortical thickness is maintained by exercise with age. Whereas this notion has not yet been tested in animals, it is consistent with the general pattern of exercise-related effects on other brain changes with age, as well as with the ability of exercise and enrichment to increase cortical thickness in adult animals (Greenough, 1984; Anderson et al., 2002).

Conclusions

Exercise-induced plasticity in the brain is widespread. It occurs in many motor areas, as well as in the hippocampus. Additionally, we know that exercise influences muscles and the cardiovascular system. For this reason, it becomes very difficult to demonstrate that exercise effects on learning rates are the result of altered mechanisms for learning as opposed to other more general responses to exercise. Data to exclude the possibility that differences in physical fitness account for different learning rates is presented in some reports on exercise effects on spatial learning, but not all potential confounds have been ruled out. For example, the ease with which the rat responds to the demand for energy during swimming could influence the cognitive resources available, or strategy chosen, to solve the task. The most convincing studies of exercise-related improvements in learning are reports that exercise affects conditioned reflexes (Baruch et al., 2004). Exercise did not influence general responses or sensitivity to stimuli, nor did it affect all types of learning. Only contextual fear conditioning, a form of conditioning dependent upon the hippocampus, was enhanced.

Earlier we stated the overall hypothesis that exercise would exert influence on the brain through increases in neural activity associated with walking and running. This hypothesis assumes that plasticity in response to exercise may be localized. Only a few studies have measured multiple regions within animals (Stummer et al., 1994; Neeper et al., 1996; Chennaoui et al., 2001; McCloskey et al., 2001; Lambert et al., 2005). The plasticity data are consistent with, although they do not confirm, the hypothesis that exercise-induced plasticity is a direct consequence of increased neural activity in individual brain structures, rather than produced solely as an indirect consequence of exercise effects on the cardiovascular and hormonal systems.

From the research reviewed, we can conclude that exercise alters many different variables within the brain. Furthermore, exercise alters many variables in a regionally selective manner. The majority of the studies reviewed were from adult but not aged animals. Although general hormonal and cardiovascular effects of exercise cannot account for all of the effects described, and therefore seem unlikely to solely account for the cognitive benefits from exercise in adult animals, it is possible that general effects may have a more prominent role in the cognitive effects seen during aging. During aging, vascular health, endocrine regulation, temperature control, and peripheral nerves all change. Thus exercise effects on specific neural systems may interact with the broader age-related changes to underlie the cognitive effects of exercise in aging. With this in mind, more research on the effects of exercise in aged animals would be helpful for understanding the mechanisms through which exercise produces cognitive benefits in this population.

CHAPTER 6

Physical Activity and Neurocognitive Function Across the Life Span

Charles H. Hillman, PhD
Department of Kinesiology and Community Health,
University of Illinois at Urbana-Champaign

Sarah M. Buck
Department of Health, Physical Education, and Recreation,
Chicago State University

Jason R. Themanson
Department of Psychology,
Illinois Wesleyan University

In recent years, there has been growing interest in the relationship between physical activity and cognition. Researchers have sought to determine the exact nature of this relationship to better understand factors that relate to increased health and effective functioning. The issue of cognitive health and function becomes especially relevant for individuals in the late stages of the human life span. A wealth of evidence now exists that demonstrates both general and selective decrements in cognition associated with advanced aging. Thus the investigation of lifestyle factors that may ameliorate or protect against cognitive loss during aging has gained interest among researchers and practitioners across a variety of health-related fields.

One aspect of cognition that is particularly amenable to physical activity intervention is executive control (see Colcombe & Kramer, 2003 for review). Researchers have outlined a number of cognitive processes that are influenced by aerobic exercise participation. Of interest, older adults exhibit disproportionate decrements in executive control relative to other types of cognition. The determination of lifestyle factors that protect against loss of executive function is particularly relevant. Accordingly, one purpose of this chapter is to review the executive control literature and describe the relationship of aging to this aspect of cognition.

Beyond behavioral measures of cognition, a growing literature base has emerged that incorporates neuroimaging to better determine the functional neuroanatomy and specific cognitive processes involved in information processing that are influenced by physical activity participation. One such measure is that of event-related brain potentials (ERPs), which index neuroelectric activation associated with specific cognitive processes. The main focus of this chapter is to examine physical activity effects on ERP indices of cognition. Although a number of other neuroimaging and behavioral techniques have been used to examine this relationship, they are beyond the scope of the chapter and therefore are not discussed in extensive detail (see Kramer & Hillman, 2006 for review of these other neuroimaging techniques).

Before turning attention to the relationship of physical activity to the brain and cognition, we provide background on the literature pertaining to executive control, cognitive aging, and the neuroelectric system to offer a rationale for why physical activity may be well suited to increasing the cognitive health and effective functioning of individuals during the late stages of the human life span. We then present an argument for providing physical activity interventions earlier in the life span, since recent evidence from our laboratory indicates that physical activity participation is related to cognitive health and function in preadolescent children. The chapter concludes with discussion on the limitations of the empirical research completed thus far and suggests several directions to guide future research efforts.

Executive Control

The term *executive control* has been used to describe a subset of processes concerned with the selection, scheduling, and coordination of the computational processes responsible for perception, memory, and action (Meyer & Keiras, 1997; Norman & Shallice, 1986). Executive processes require conscious awareness, are functionally distinct from processes they organize, and are limited in their resources (Rogers & Monsell, 1995). Because of these characteristics, tasks requiring executive processes do not habituate or become automatic over time.

One proposed theoretical model of executive control (Norman & Shallice, 1986) assumes a top-down approach to cognitive processing and action execution. This model suggests that multiple subsystems interact and are under the control of two distinct mechanisms: contention scheduling and the supervisory attentional system (SAS). Contention scheduling is the lower-order level of control, which automatically selects action schemas to execute well-learned processes that are active until goal attainment or inhibition by a competing schema or supervisory control. Thus, adoption of the appropriate response to a task (i.e., a task-set or action schema) does not typically involve the intervention of the executive mechanism. In most instances, the suitable task-set can be automatically selected through the contention scheduling process. However, in some instances an action schema or task-set may not be available to achieve control of the desired behavior, especially when tasks are novel or complex. On these occasions, additional control is provided through the SAS (Norman & Shallice, 1986). The SAS operates by providing increased inhibition or activation to competing schemas to bias the selection of schemas through the contention scheduling mechanism. In this manner, the individual's component processes can be reorganized to meet the current demands and objectives of the task. Thus, the SAS is an attentional control process that modulates, biases, or even restarts the selection process and is primarily related to the initiation rather than the execution of action (Norman & Shallice, 1986).

Cognitive Control

Within the framework of executive control is the online implementation of one's thoughts, actions, and emotions, which is often referred to as cognitive control. That is, cognitive control is a subset of executive processes responsible for adjustments in perceptual selection, biasing of responses, and online maintenance of contextual information (Botvinick et al., 2001). Thus, cognitive control processes are often associated with a "central executive" in theoretical models. This executive is responsible for the adaptability of the cognitive system and is often specified similarly to the SAS (Baddeley, 1996; Norman & Shallice, 1986).

However, cognitive control processes are not unitary; and the adaptability of the cognitive system needs to be understood not only in terms of what increases control influences in an individual's interaction with the environment, but also in terms of how increased control is implemented or brought about to intervene under the appropriate circumstances. To address these issues, researchers have suggested that there are at least two functionally linked but dissociable systems of cognitive control, termed evaluative and regulative (see Botvinick et al., 2001 for review).

The evaluative system of cognitive control monitors for instances of conflict during information-processing events. More specifically, the evaluative system detects the occurrence of conflict during cognitive processing and sends signals to processing centers responsible for providing compensatory adjustments of top-down control that are necessary for successful adaptations to task demands (Botvinick et al., 2001). Neuroimaging research has suggested that the anterior cingulate cortex (ACC) is involved in the evaluative system and the signaling and detection of conflict. Most notably, results indicate that ACC activation is largest when cognitive control is weak (Botvinick et al., 1999; Carter et al., 2000). Further, increased ACC activation in conjunction with weak cognitive control may indicate the signaling for adjustments in control to more strongly engage the strategic processes necessary for improvements in subsequent behavior (MacDonald et al., 2000).

The regulative system exerts top-down control during ongoing information processing. That is, flexible adjustments in strategic support are provided for task-relevant interactions within the stimulus environment, allowing for improved representations and active attentional maintenance of task demands. Available neuroimaging research indicates that this regulative support is likely provided, at least in part, by the dorsolateral prefrontal cortex (DLPFC; MacDonald et al., 2000). Thus, the two components of cognitive control interact as part of a negative feedback loop to optimize performance (MacDonald et al., 2000). In this loop, the DLPFC implements cognitive control for task-related behaviors; the ACC monitors for conflict during task execution and signals for the increased engagement of control in instances of conflict; and the DLPFC responds to signals of conflict with an adaptive adjustment to upregulate control in an attempt to improve subsequent behavioral interactions with the environment.

Cognitive Aging

With aging come changes in brain structure and function. Coupled with these age-related changes in the neurobiology are changes in cognitive functions associated with the affected brain structures. Responsible for changes in brain structure are well-documented age-related reductions in brain volume and ventricular enlargement (Davis & Wright, 1977). Brain volume reductions are due to reductions in the volume of gray matter (Salat et al., 2004). However, reductions in white matter volume, related to decreases in the number of synapses and the atrophy of dendritic processes, are also evident with advancing age (West, 1996). Changes in neurotransmitter function have also been observed with age. Recent evidence suggests that these age-related decrements begin during early adulthood, with an acceleration of loss occurring during later adulthood (Fotenos et al., 2005). Although age-related decrements have been observed across multiple brain structures (Raz, 2000), substantial decrements in two distinct anatomical circuits have been identified. The first involves the frontal cortex and basal ganglia, and the other involves the hippocampal formation and related medial temporal lobe structures (Buckner, Head, & Lustig, 2006). Accordingly, functions subserved by these brain structures have been found to be especially susceptible to cognitive aging.

Relative to young adults, older adults exhibit performance deficits across a wide variety of tasks that tap a number of cognitive processes including visuospatial and verbal memory (Park et al., 2002), working memory (Hasher & Zacks, 1988), long-term memory (Zacks & Hasher, 2006), attention (Kramer & Kray, 2006), and executive control (Kramer et al., 1994), among other cognitive functions. Thus it appears that age-related changes in brain structure and function lead to general decrements in cognition during later stages of the life span. However, Kramer and his colleagues (1994) have indicated that cognitive aging is not unitary, as disproportionately larger deficits in cognitive performance have been found for tasks or task components requiring greater amounts of executive control. Further, certain executive functions are more susceptible to age-related decline than others. Given that the frontal lobe also exhibits a disproportionate loss of function relative to other brain regions (Haug & Eggers, 1991), it is not surprising that processes mediated by this region of the cortex would evidence disproportionate loss during aging. Dempster (1992) reviewed the role of the frontal lobes in cognitive development and stated that they are among the earliest to show signs of deterioration due to age, with that area of brain tissue characterized by a significant decrease in blood flow, weight, and cortical thickness during the later stages of the life span.

Specifically, Kramer and his colleagues (Kramer, Hahn, & Gopher, 1999; Kramer et al., 1994) used several tests of executive control (e.g., task-switching, Wisconsin Card Sorting Task, negative priming, response compatibility, stopping) to further understand the effects of aging on inhibitory processes. Their findings indicated that older, compared to younger, adults exhibited decreased performance (i.e., reaction time [RT], error rate) on certain tasks (e.g., response compatibility, stopping) but were equivalent for other tasks (e.g., negative compatibility), indicating that age-related decrements in executive control are not unitary. The authors interpreted their findings by suggesting that age-related deficits in performance are specific to certain failures in inhibitory processes rather than a more general failure in overall inhibitory control. Interestingly, the tasks that elicited the largest age-related performance differences were those that are mediated, in large part, by the frontal lobes, whereas the tasks in which aging differences were not observed were mediated by other regions of the brain. This would suggest that aging might specifically compromise inhibitory processes mediated by the frontal lobe (Kramer et al., 1994).

Although a wealth of other data also point to selectively larger age-related decrements for (executive) tasks subserved by the frontal lobe, the purpose of this chapter is not to provide an exhaustive review of cognitive aging. However, germane to the chapter is that cognitive performance decreases during later stages of the life span, and further, that tasks mediated by specific brain regions exhibit disproportionately larger decrements. Accordingly, one guiding framework for the literature examining physical activity effects on cognitive aging as described here is that tasks (or task components) engaging the frontal lobe may be especially responsive to lifestyle factors that promote increased health and function, compared to tasks that are mediated by other brain regions and exhibit fewer signs of cognitive aging. The body of research we describe is limited in scope to the neuroelectric system. Compared to a growing literature base addressing general and selective physical activity effects on cognitive function (see Colcombe & Kramer, 2003 for review), the literature base on the neuroelectric system remains considerably smaller. Accordingly, the goal of this chapter is to provide a detailed review of the relationship between physical activity participation and neuroelectric concomitants of cognition during performance of tasks that require variable amounts of executive control, thus allowing for greater understanding of the general and selective influence of physical activity on cognitive aging.

Neuroelectric Measurement

Electroencephalographic (EEG) activity is a recording of the difference in electrical potentials between various locations on the scalp. When electrodes are placed on the scalp, the EEG reflects activity of large populations of neurons firing in sync (Hugdahl, 1995). The dipoles from the individual neurons must be spatially aligned perpendicular to the scalp in order to be detected (Luck, 2005). Thus, EEG measurement is most likely to result from cortical pyramidal cells, which are aligned perpendicular to the cortex surface (Luck, 2005). This type of measurement has long been used to assess cognition and more recently to identify potential physiological mechanisms underlying the beneficial relationship between fitness and cognition. In particular, ERPs, which are a class of EEG activity, appear to be susceptible to the effects of exercise (Polich & Lardon, 1997), and refer to fluctuations in neuroelectric activity that are related to the occurrence of a stimulus or event. Event-related potentials may be classified as either exogenous (i.e., obligatory responses dependent upon the physical properties of the eliciting stimulus) or endogenous (i.e., higher-order cognitive processes that often require active participation from the subject, but are independent of the physical properties of the stimulus environment). Given the direction of previous research on physical activity and neurocognition, this chapter focuses solely on endogenous components of an ERP.

Stimulus-locked ERP components are named based on their polarity (i.e., negative or positive deflections of the waveform) and ordinal position along the waveform. The typical ERP to a visual stimulus consists of a complex of several components, with earlier components (P1, N1, P2) relating to aspects of spatial attention and later components (N2, P3 or P3b) relating to various facets of cognitive function (e.g., detection of deviant stimuli, working memory; Luck, 2005). For more extensive descriptions of the stimulus-locked ERP components, the interested reader is referred to a review by Coles and Rugg (1995).

Response-locked components, including the error-related negativity (ERN) and the error positivity (Pe), are thought to be related to neural correlates of action monitoring and error awareness, respectively. The ERN is a negative deflection of the waveform at frontal and central electrode sites that begins just after an incorrect response is made. The Pe is a positive deflection of the waveform at centroparietal sites occurring approximately 300 ms after an incorrect response. Physical activity, fitness, or both appear to relate to changes in various components of an ERP waveform, including the P3, ERN, and Pe.

Having provided a rationale for the need to better understand factors that may ameliorate or protect against cognitive aging, as well as a brief description of disproportionate loss of executive control during older adulthood, in the remainder of the chapter we examine the relationship between physical activity and neurocognition. We specifically focus on the neuroelectric system by first reviewing the literature on stimulus-locked ERPs and then the literature on response-locked ERPs. Finally, we discuss extensions of this work to cognitive development.

Physical Activity Influences on Stimulus-Locked ERPs

In this section we focus on the P3 component (also known as the P300 or P3b), which has been examined most commonly in studies using simple discrimination tasks. The neuroelectric literature has provided strong support for age-related deficits in the expression of P3. In adult populations, however, a number of studies have demonstrated a positive relationship between physical activity and decreased P3 latency, as well as between physical activity and increased P3 amplitude.

The P3 Component

The P3 is a positive deflection in an ERP (Sutton et al., 1965) that peaks approximately 300 to 1000 ms after stimulus onset, depending on task complexity and individual characteristics in the sample tested. Because of its relation to aspects of information processing, this endogenous component has captured considerable attention in the literature. Although the P3 may be recorded using a variety of tasks and paradigms, it has most commonly been elicited by simple discrimination tasks, such as an oddball task in which individuals must discriminate between two stimuli that are presented in a long and random series. The participants' task is to respond to one or to both stimuli, which occur with differing probabilities (see Polich, 2004 for review).

The precise neural tissue mediating the P3 response is unknown, since this ERP component likely reflects a network of neural circuitry and generators. However, discrimination tasks requiring attentional focus are thought to elicit frontal lobe activation (Posner, 1992; Posner & Petersen, 1990), with ERP (i.e., P3a) and functional magnetic resonance imaging (fMRI) studies demonstrating greater frontal lobe activity in response to rare or alerting stimuli (Polich, 2004). The ACC is activated when working memory representations of the stimulus environment change, which in turn signals the inferotemporal lobe for stimulus maintenance (i.e., memory storage). The P3 (i.e., P3b) component is elicited when attentional resources are allocated for subsequent memory updating after stimulus evaluation. This is thought to occur when memory storage operations initiated in the hippocampal formation are transmitted to the parietal cortex, which is typically where the P3 exhibits maximal amplitude in the scalp distribution (Squire & Kandell, 1999; Knight, 1996). Thus, the neuroelectric events that underlie P3 generation occur from the interaction between frontal lobe and hippocampal/temporal-parietal function (Knight, 1996; Polich, 2004) to modulate attentional control over the contents of working memory (Polich, 2004).

The P3 has been examined extensively in order to investigate aspects of information processing related to stimulus engagement. That is, the P3 has been hypothesized to represent the allocation of attentional resources involved in working memory operations during context updating of the stimulus environment once sensory information has been analyzed (Donchin, 1981; Donchin & Coles, 1988). The amplitude of the P3 component is thought to reflect changes in the neural representation of the stimulus environment and is proportional to the amount of attentional resources needed to engage a given stimulus or task, with greater attentional allocation increasing P3 amplitude (Polich & Heine, 1996). The latency of the P3 component is a measure of stimulus evaluation or cognitive processing speed (Duncan-Johnson, 1981), with longer latencies reflecting increased processing time.

Decreases in P3 amplitude elicited during paradigms with short interstimulus intervals have been observed during tasks or task conditions requiring more extensive amounts of executive control. For example, smaller P3 amplitude has been found during the incongruent, relative to the congruent, condition for a flanker task in both younger and older adults (Hillman et al., 2004; Hillman, Snook, & Jerome, 2003); this is due to the increased need for interference control in the incongruent condition and additional demands placed upon the recovery cycle that underlie the mechanisms responsible for generation of the P3 component (Gonsalvez & Polich, 2002). In a flanker task, participants are required to discriminate between target stimuli that are flanked by an array of other stimuli with which different responses are associated. Differences in response accuracy and speed are observed between congruent (e.g., HHHHH) and incongruent (e.g., HHSHH) conditions, with the former eliciting faster and more accurate responses than the latter (Eriksen & Schultz, 1979). The incongruent task requires greater amounts of interference control (one aspect of executive control) to inhibit task-irrelevant stimuli and execute the correct response. Specifically, the flanking stimuli activate the incorrect response to the task, which competes with the correct response elicited by the centrally placed target stimulus (Spencer & Coles, 1999).

Other research has evidenced topographic differences in P3 amplitude during a Go/NoGo task, which manipulates stimulus probability and requires variable amounts of response inhibition, with maximal amplitude observed parietally during the Go condition and frontocentrally during the NoGo condition (Tekok-Kilic, Shucard, & Shucard, 2001). Given that the NoGo condition requires greater amounts of inhibitory control due to the need to suppress a prepotent motor response, these findings again suggest that P3 amplitude is sensitive to task conditions requiring variable amounts of executive control. Further, the findings reflect deficits or inefficiencies (i.e., decreased amplitude or shifts in scalp topography) in neuroelectric resource allocation associated with attention during tasks that have larger executive control requirements. P3 latency may also be used to index neurocognitive deficits in information processing during executive control operations, as longer P3 latency has been observed during task components with greater executive requirements in older and younger adults (Hillman et al., 2004, 2006). This robust finding indicates that P3 latency measures alterations in cognitive processing speed associated with task requirements, and suggests decreases in the efficiency of the neuroelectric system during tasks necessitating greater amounts of executive control (Hillman et al., 2006; Zeef et al., 1996). Given these findings, the P3 is considered a useful tool for understanding covert alterations in information processing, even in the absence of changes in overt performance across experimental manipulations.

Aging and P3

One of the most robust findings in the neuroelectric literature is age-related deficits in the expression of the P3 component (Fabiani & Friedman, 1995; Fabiani, Friedman, & Cheng, 1998; Picton et al., 1984; Polich, 1997). Picton and colleagues (1984) used auditory stimuli to elicit the P3 from participants of different age groups (20-79 years, 12 participants from each decade). P3 amplitude declined with age at a rate of 0.18 μV/year, and the scalp distribution became more frontal due to age-related decreases in amplitude at the vertex of the scalp. Thus the observed similarity across electrode sites on the scalp that accompany aging may relate to an inefficiency of neuroelectric processes underlying cognitive function. Other researchers have used dipole modeling techniques to localize the neural generators of the P3, with results supporting increased frontal lobe involvement during aging (Friedman, Simpson, & Hamberger, 1993). This finding suggests that older adults may exert greater amounts of executive control during tasks that do not normally require extensive top-down executive control support in younger individuals. Accordingly, age-related decrements in the cognitive processes indexed by P3 scalp distribution are suggestive of alterations in neurobiological integrity. That is, the observed similarity across electrode sites on the scalp that accompany aging may relate to the decreased efficiency of these processes. Given that there is an overall reduction of P3 amplitude for older compared to younger adults, one might speculate that the increased similarity observed in the topographic distribution is indicative of some compensatory mechanism that helps older adults meet the demands of the imposed challenge. These aging differences would be expected to emerge more frequently when greater amounts of executive control (which has been shown to be subserved by the frontal lobe) are required.

Brain lesion data further support the differential activation of the frontal lobe during aging. Specifically, Knight (1984, 1997) used common (frequent, ignored), rare (required participant response), and novel (uninstructed, task irrelevant) stimuli to examine differences in scalp distribution between patients with lesions in the DLPFC and nonlesion controls. Results indicated that during the novelty condition, control participants exhibited frontally distributed P3 responses compared to lesion patients, who showed parietally distributed P3 responses. Since the DLPFC has been implicated in orienting behavior (Luria, 1973), Knight's findings suggest that the DLPFC is involved in the modulation or generation of novelty P3 (i.e., P3a). Further, these data support the importance of the frontal lobe in stimulus evaluation processes, suggesting that if these regions are compromised during advanced aging, biases in stimulus engagement and response selection may occur.

With regard to the latency of P3, Picton and colleagues (1984) reported an increase of 1.36 ms/year beginning in early adulthood. Other laboratories have corroborated these results and found similar latency decrements (O'Donnell et al., 1992). O'Donnell and his colleagues (1992) suggested that cognitive processing speed, measured via P3 latency, contributes to decreased task performance (e.g., RT) of older individuals. P3 latency measured during a flanker task, which manipulated interference control requirements, was longer for older compared to younger participants and for the incongruent relative to the congruent condition. However, latency differences for age and congruency did not interact, suggesting that age-related decrements in processing speed during tasks that require interference control may not be related to stimulus evaluation; rather, age-related differences may be due to other ongoing executive processes (Zeef et al., 1996). Taken together, the cognitive aging data regarding the P3 component indicate deficits in the allocation of neuroelectric resources in terms of the amount and topography of the amplitude, as well as the speed at which cognitive processing occurs during stimulus engagement. As such, these age-related deficits in cognitive function increase the reliance upon executive control operations, even when characteristics of the stimulus environment would not normally require such top-down control during earlier periods of the adult life span.

Physical Activity and the P3 Component in Adult Populations

Currently, an abundance of evidence indicates that physical activity, and aerobic exercise in particular, benefits cognition on the cellular, systems, and behavioral levels, with research showing that cognitive function of older adults is especially amenable to physical activity intervention (Colcombe & Kramer, 2003; Bashore, 1989; Dustman et al., 1990; Kramer et al., 1999). Habitual participation in aerobic exercise, which leads to improvements in cardiorespiratory fitness, has been found to decrease neuroelectric performance differences between older and younger adults, indicating that exercise may help to maintain overall cognitive health (Dustman, Shearer, & Emmerson, 1993; Hillman et al., 2002, 2004, 2006).

P3 Latency

Some of the earliest research examining aerobic exercise effects on ERPs was performed by Dustman and his colleagues (Dustman et al., 1985, 1990), who observed that P3 latency was faster in aerobically trained compared to sedentary older males performing an oddball task. The reduction was great enough to lead to nonsignificant differences between the older fit males and younger adults, whereas older sedentary males exhibited significantly longer P3 latencies. These data indicated that aerobic exercise improved cognitive processing speed or protected against age-related decrements in processing speed in older men. Other researchers have corroborated or extended Dustman's findings using tasks with small executive control requirements (Bashore, 1989; Hillman et al., 2002).

Given the recent findings of disproportionately larger age-related deficits in executive control processes that are subserved by the frontal lobe, the relationship of physical activity to these processes is of great interest from the viewpoint of determining means for protecting against cognitive aging and maintaining cognitive health during the later stages of the life span. Accordingly, Hillman and colleagues (2004, 2006) used various executive control tasks to determine the relationship between physical activity and neurocognitive performance during older adulthood. Findings indicated that greater amounts of physical activity were associated with faster P3 latency (Hillman et al., 2004, 2006). From these studies, two important findings were obtained. First, greater amounts of aerobic activity in older adults were related to linear decreases in P3 latency. Specifically, faster latency was observed for high-active older adults relative to their moderate- and low-active peers (Hillman et al., 2004). Secondly, the relationship between physical activity and P3 latency is selectively greater for task components requiring greater amounts of executive control (Hillman et al., 2006). That is, during task conditions requiring individuals to hold two rule sets in working memory and flexibly shift between rule sets, high-active individuals exhibited faster P3 latency than low-active individuals. However, during task conditions requiring individuals to hold only one rule set in working memory without the need to shift between sets, no physical activity–related differences were observed (Hillman et al., 2006). Taken together, these findings indicate the disproportionately larger relationship between physical activity and cognitive processing speed during executive control tasks and suggest a linear relationship between physical activity participation and benefits in older adults' processing speed.

P3 Amplitude

In addition to improvements in cognitive processing speed, physical activity has been related to differential allocation of neuroelectric resources during older adulthood. Most notably, active individuals exhibit increased P3 amplitude when compared to their sedentary counterparts, and these findings are indicative of greater allocation of attentional resources with physical activity participation. Early researchers employed oddball (Polich & Lardon, 1997) and other speeded perceptual (Bashore, 1989) tasks to examine physical activity effects on P3 amplitude, with results indicating a positive relationship. More recent investigations have corroborated these findings (McDowell et al., 2003) and extended them to include somatosensory oddball tasks in which participants received electrical stimulation to their index fingers (Hatta et al., 2005). Importantly, Hatta and colleagues (2005) also observed greater heterogeneity across midline scalp sites for high-active, relative to low-active, older participants, suggesting greater specificity of neuroelectric resource allocation with increased amounts of physical activity. However, other research has failed to examine physical activity effects on P3 amplitude in older adults using simple stimulus discrimination tasks (Dustman et al., 1990; Hillman et al., 2002).

On the basis of the inconsistent findings indicating that physical activity either has a positive effect on or is unrelated to P3 amplitude and its topographic distribution during older adulthood, research in our laboratory has been aimed at determining whether the relation of physical activity to P3 (and the processes subsumed by it) would be more robust when examined within the context of tasks that are dependent upon the frontal lobe, since this region of the brain exhibits a disproportionate loss of structure and function during aging. As described previously in connection with P3 latency, we conducted two studies that used task conditions requiring variable amounts of executive control. Both studies included older and younger participants so that we could determine not only the influence of physical activity participation on P3, but also whether the relationship changes with age during adulthood. As predicted, higher-active older adults exhibited increased P3 amplitude at electrode sites over the frontal region of the scalp (Hillman et al., 2004, 2006). Specifically, moderate- and high-active older adults had larger P3 amplitude relative to younger adults during tasks requiring greater amounts of executive control (i.e., incongruent flanker conditions that necessitate greater interference control). This relationship was not observed for low-active older participants, and no such effect was observed during task conditions requiring smaller amounts of interference control (Hillman et al., 2004). These findings suggest that physical activity is associated with increased allocation of attentional resources during task performance, and that this relationship is selectively greater during tasks that necessitate increases in frontally mediated executive control function.

Additional support for these findings was obtained using a task-switching paradigm, which as described previously manipulates working memory load and requires cognitive flexibility during switching between rule sets. The comparison of older and younger adults who varied in their physical activity participation corroborated our earlier efforts (Hillman et al., 2004) and extended them to an additional aspect of executive control. In particular, older active adults exhibited larger P3 amplitude over frontally placed scalp sites relative to their sedentary peers and to both physically active and sedentary younger adult groups. However, shifts in scalp topography were observed that were dependent upon both age and physical activity participation, such that both older and younger active participants exhibited larger P3 amplitude than their sedentary peers at central scalp sites. Further, younger active participants exhibited larger amplitude over parietal scalp sites relative to the other three groups. Given that younger adults exhibited the classic and robust P3 topography, which includes a parietal maximum (i.e., P3 amplitude is largest over parietal scalp sites), the increase in P3 amplitude for high-active older adults may reflect compensatory neural function during stimulus engagement to improve or maintain task performance. Task performance data supported this hypothesis, as faster RTs were observed for physically active relative to sedentary participants, regardless of age. Additional support was garnered from the sedentary participants, who exhibited smaller amplitude and decreased heterogeneity of scalp topography, which indicated smaller and less efficient allocation of neuroelectric resources during a task requiring variable amounts of executive control.

Data from these two studies reveal that physical activity may benefit a subset of processes involved in information processing that occur between stimulus engagement and response production. Further, the influence of physical activity on these neuroelectric processes appears to benefit the allocation and efficiency of cognitive processing in this system and has implications for task performance. Taken together, these findings suggest that physical activity may help to ameliorate or protect against cognitive aging, and they support physical activity as a potential mediator for cognitive aging. Lastly, the data also indicate that physical activity is beneficial to cognition during young adulthood, suggesting that the adoption of a physically active lifestyle may be associated with improved cognitive health and function during earlier stages of the life span.

Physical Activity Influences on Response-Locked ERPS

In this section we look at research that has addressed the influence of physical activity and fitness on action monitoring and error correction processes and their neural correlates, the ERN and the Pe. The ERN appears to be more efficient in physically active compared to sedentary older adults, and higher-fit individuals exhibit both smaller ERN amplitude and larger Pe amplitude than individuals with lower levels of fitness.

Action Monitoring

People are typically aware of the consequences of their actions. Specifically, when individuals make an incorrect judgment or an error in a cognitive task, they often have an awareness of the error and react out of frustration in a visible or audible way (Yeung, Cohen, & Botvinick, 2004). Further, the participant is often able to express that an error was made by consequently exhibiting the appropriate response (Rabbitt, 1966). According to Rabbitt (2002), this explicit detection and specification of the error is mostly accurate (79% of errors are detected by young adults) and often deliberate and effortful (700 ms latency following error commission). However, behavioral correction of an error is fast and relatively automatic (Yeung, Cohen, & Botvinick, 2004). Participants are able to produce a corrective response (i.e., the response they initially should have made to complete the task correctly) anywhere between 20 ms (Rabbitt, Cumming, & Vyas, 1978) and 250 ms (Rabbitt, 2002) following the error response. Thus, errors provide individuals with an important source of information in relation to their subsequent interaction with the environment and the corrective actions or processes that need to occur for performance to improve. These corrective actions can be fast and automatic, or they can be more deliberate and related to conscious recognition of error commission.

These behavioral findings and the related investigation of action monitoring and error correction processes have gained interest in recent years with the discovery of neural correlates of action monitoring. In particular, studies of ERPs have revealed neural indices of both fast and relatively automatic action monitoring processes (i.e., ERN) and corrective action monitoring processes that are more deliberate and related to error awareness (i.e., Pe).

Error-Related Negativity

One neural response following error commission is the error-related negativity (ERN: Gehring et al., 1993; or Ne: Falkenstein et al., 1991). The ERN is a negative-going component observed in response-locked ERP averages of incorrect responses. It is maximal over frontocentral recording sites and peaks shortly after incorrect responses in speeded RT tasks (Falkenstein et al., 1991; Gehring et al., 1993). The ERN has been shown to be evident regardless of an individual's awareness of error commission (Nieuwenhuis et al., 2001), and it is reduced following error responses to infrequent stimuli (Holroyd & Coles, 2002). Further, researchers have localized the source of the ERN at or very near the dorsal ACC using dipole localization techniques (Dehaene, Posner, & Tucker, 1994; van Veen & Carter, 2002), and corroborating evidence has come from both neuroimaging (Carter et al., 1998) and magnetoencephalography studies (Miltner et al., 2003). Neuroimaging findings have established that the functional significance of ACC activation is related to action monitoring and evaluation during tasks requiring extensive executive control (Carter et al., 2000). Further, Gehring and Knight (2000) have shown that the ACC exhibits a functional interaction with the prefrontal cortex during action monitoring processes and compensatory or corrective actions following error responses.

Though the ERN is generally believed to reflect a cognitive learning mechanism used to correct an individual's responses during subsequent environmental interactions, the specific functional significance of the ERN remains unresolved. Two distinct theories have suggested differential processes that relate to ERN activation. One theory holds that the ERN measures error detection and monitoring (Berstein, Scheffers, & Coles, 1995; Falkenstein et al., 1991; Scheffers et al., 1996). More specifically, this reinforcement learning model (Holroyd & Coles, 2002) proposes that the ERN is part of a system that detects the occurrence of an error and uses that information to improve task performance. The ERN is evidenced on error trials through a reduction in dopaminergic activity that disinhibits the ACC, which in turn selects the appropriate motor controllers to successfully complete the task based upon this input (Holroyd & Coles, 2002).

An alternative theory suggests that the ERN reflects a conflict monitoring process (Botvinick et al., 2001). This process is part of a system involving the ACC that detects (or monitors) levels of response conflict. This information is then transmitted from the ACC to processing control centers, which triggers adjustments in relative influences on processing among the control centers (Botvinick et al., 2001). Although the true function of the ERN is debated, there is consensus that the ACC is the primary structure driving the ERN signal (Carter et al., 1998; Miltner et al., 2003).

Error Positivity

A second ERP component related to action monitoring processes following error responses is the error positivity (Pe: Falkenstein et al., 1990, 2000). The Pe is a positive-going component observed in response-locked ERP averages of incorrect responses. It is maximal over centroparietal recording sites and peaks after the ERN (about 300 ms following an incorrect response). Further, research using dipole localization techniques has identified generators of the Pe in the rostral ACC (van Veen & Carter, 2002). Although both the ERN and Pe are associated with neural processes in the ACC, the two components have distinct neural generators and are believed to be independent of each other (Herrmann et al., 2004).

The Pe has been described as an emotional reaction to the commission of an error (Falkenstein et al., 2000; van Veen & Carter, 2002), as a postresponse evaluation of an error (Davies et al., 2001; Falkenstein et al., 1990), and as the allocation of attentional resources toward an error following error commission (Mathewson, Dywan, & Segalowitz, 2005). More specifically, Davies and colleagues (2001) found strong correlations between Pe and P3 amplitude, suggesting that the Pe could be a P3-like response to the internal detection of an error, with the error response being the salient stimulus to which attentional resources are allocated. Additionally, Mathewson and coworkers (2005) found that both increased P3 and Pe amplitudes were associated with better task performance (i.e., fewer errors) across multiple cognitive tasks, though these relationships were different across age groupings. The finding of an association between increased Pe amplitude and improved task performance has been verified independently (Falkenstein et al., 2000) and provides support for the notion that the Pe may be a neuroelectric index of compensatory actions following the commission of an error through the increase of attentional control (Themanson & Hillman, 2006).

Physical Activity and Action Monitoring

Currently, only two published studies have addressed physical activity and fitness in relation to response-locked ERPs. The initial study (Themanson, Hillman, & Curtin, 2006) assessed the relationship between self-reported physical activity behavior, ERN amplitude, and posterror behavior for 53 older and younger adults during a task requiring variable amounts of executive control (i.e., task-switching) in which participants were instructed to respond as quickly as possible. Physical activity was assessed using the

Yale Physical Activity Survey for Older Adults (YPAS; DiPietro et al., 1993), which measures activities of daily living and comprises three subscales: total hours of activity, kilocalorie expenditure, and the Yale Summary Index (YSI). The YSI estimates the average amount of physical activity during the previous month and is highly correlated with $\dot{V}O_2$peak in older adults (Young, Jee, & Appel, 2001). The results from this initial study indicated that older adults exhibited a greater relative slowing in RT during switch blocks and smaller ERN amplitude compared to younger adults; both of these findings corroborated previous aging research.

However, physical activity differences were also observed that revealed a relatively smaller switch cost (i.e., RT on switch trials – RT on nonswitch trials) for physically active older adults, indicating better performance during tasks that place an increased load on working memory. Further, decreased ERN amplitude for older and younger physically active participants and relatively greater response slowing following commission of errors were observed when compared with values for the sedentary counterparts (Themanson, Hillman, & Curtin, 2006). Given that posterror response slowing is a behavioral indicator of increased recruitment and implementation of top-down attentional control to improve performance on subsequent environmental interactions (Gehring et al., 1993; Kerns et al., 2004), these findings suggest increased attentional control among physically active individuals regardless of age (Themanson, Hillman, & Curtin, 2006). This increase in top-down attentional control not only improves behavioral performance, but also decreases the activation associated with the evaluative component of action monitoring processes during speeded task performance. Thus, the resulting neuroelectric signal (i.e., ERN) indicative of response monitoring may be described as more efficient in physically active adults, and may relate to increases in top-down adjustments used to correct behavior following error commission.

Fitness and Action Monitoring

A second study examined the influence of cardiorespiratory fitness on ERP components related to action monitoring, using two groups of young adults that exhibited large differences in their respective levels of fitness (Themanson & Hillman, 2006). The study focused on neuroelectric (i.e., ERN, Pe) and behavioral (i.e., posterror slowing) indices of action monitoring processes acquired during the completion of a flanker task in which 28 higher- and lower-fit young adult participants were required to respond as quickly as possible. Participants completed a graded exercise test to assess their level of cardiorespiratory fitness through measurement of maximal oxygen consumption ($\dot{V}O_2$max). Additionally, cognitive testing was conducted for each individual on two separate, and counterbalanced, occasions: once after a 30 min period of rest and once after a 30 min bout of hard but submaximal (83.5% maximal heart rate) treadmill exercise (Themanson & Hillman, 2006). Findings demonstrated a relationship between levels of cardiorespiratory fitness and indices of action monitoring such that the higher-fit group exhibited smaller ERN amplitude than the lower-fit group, suggesting a relative reduction in the conflict-related neuroelectric index of action monitoring associated with error responses. Additionally, higher-fit individuals exhibited both larger Pe amplitude and greater posterror response slowing than lower-fit individuals, which indicated an increase in both neural and behavioral posterror adjustments in top-down attentional control.

Together, these two studies indicate that individuals with greater levels of fitness or physical activity participation are exerting increased levels of top-down attentional control during task execution. This increase in top-down attentional control is associated with a reduced activation of the neuroelectric system designed to respond to indicants of task performance conflicts, resulting in an overall reduced ERN amplitude (Themanson & Hillman, 2006; Themanson, Hillman, & Curtin, 2006). Finally, given current views of posterror slowing as a behavioral indicator of the implementation of top-down attentional control (Gehring et al., 1993; Kerns et al., 2004), and of Pe amplitude as a neuroelectric index of postresponse evaluation of an error (Davies et al., 2001; Falkenstein et al., 1990) or the allocation of attentional resources toward an error (Mathewson et al., 2005), Themanson and Hillman (2006) have argued that this increase in top-down attentional control is associated with an increased corrective response following error commission, through the observed increase in both posterror slowing and Pe amplitudes for higher-fit individuals.

The observed reductions in ERN amplitude and increase in Pe amplitude with greater levels of fitness or physical activity involvement corroborate research on the relationship between aerobic training and ACC activation (Colcombe et al., 2004). Using neuroimaging measures, Colcombe and colleagues (2004) found that aerobically trained older adults, compared to nonaerobically trained control participants, evidenced greater activation of task-related prefrontal and parietal brain regions involved with inhibitory functioning. This increase in the recruitment of relevant brain regions for higher-fit individuals suggests "an increase in the ability of the frontal attentional circuitry to bias task-related activation in posterior regions of cortex" (Colcombe et al., 2004, p. 3320), which might be indicative of an increase in Pe amplitude.

Further, reduced ACC activation was observed for aerobically trained older adults compared to their sedentary counterparts, suggesting a decrease in behavioral conflict for these individuals (Colcombe et al., 2004). This finding strongly suggests a reduction in ERN amplitude for aerobically fit individuals according to the conflict monitoring hypothesis proposed by

Botvinick and colleagues (2001). The reinforcement learning model of ERN activation (Holroyd & Coles, 2002) might also predict a relative reduction in ERN amplitude for individuals with greater levels of cardiorespiratory fitness. According to this model, a phasic reduction in dopaminergic activity is associated with the modulation of ERN amplitude. Interestingly, both animal and human studies have shown that regular aerobic exercise leads to increases in dopaminergic activity (Farrell et al., 1986; Gullestad et al., 1997; MacRae et al., 1987; Meeusen et al., 1997; Van Loon, Schwartz, & Sole, 1979; but see also Wang et al., 2000), which, according to this model, would suggest that aerobic fitness may be associated with a relative decrease in ERN amplitude through increased inhibition of the ACC.

Physical Activity Influences on Neurocognitive Function During Preadolescent Development

Given that a positive relationship has been established between fitness and cognition in older adults (see Colcombe & Kramer, 2003 for review), more attention has begun to shift toward the investigation of a similar relationship between fitness and cognitive health during earlier periods of the human life span. Preliminary findings in school-aged children indicate a comparable relationship (Sibley & Etnier, 2003), although gaps in the literature exist regarding the particular types of cognition affected and the mechanisms underlying such findings. With an increasing percentage of children living an inactive lifestyle, a greater understanding of the benefits of fitness for cognition during this period of the life span is both timely and relevant.

Sibley and Etnier (2003) conducted a meta-analysis on the relationship between physical activity and cognition in school-aged children. Forty-four studies that differed in design (i.e., true, quasi-, cross-sectional), age of participants (4-18), type of physical activity behavior (i.e., acute, chronic), training characteristics (i.e., resistance, aerobic, perceptual-motor, physical education program), and cognitive assessment (i.e., perceptual skills, intelligent quotient, achievement, verbal tests, math tests, memory, developmental level or academic readiness, and other) were included in the analyses. A significant positive relationship between physical activity and cognition was found, such that increased physical activity was related to cognitive performance along the eight measurement categories; the relationship was beneficial in all categories (Sibley & Etnier, 2003). Although this relationship was seen across all age groups, it was stronger for children in the 4- to 7- and 11- to 13-year-old groups compared to the 8- to 10- and 14- to 18-year-old groups (Sibley & Etnier, 2003).

In order to better understand some of the potential mechanisms underlying the cognitive improvements observed in children, Hillman, Castelli, and Buck (2005) examined neuroelectric indices (P3-ERP) of attentional allocation during a visual oddball task. Neuroelectric data were collected on 51 higher- and lower-fit (n = 12-15 per group, approximately equal male-to-female ratio per group) preadolescent children (M = 9.5 years, SD = 0.9 years) and young adults (M = 19.3 years, SD = 1.4 years). Participants were screened for aerobic capacity using the Progressive Aerobic Cardiovascular Endurance Run (PACER) subtest of the *Fitnessgram* (Welk, Morris, & Falls, 2002), which is a field test that assesses aerobic, strength, and flexibility fitness. Cognitive function was measured using ERPs and behavioral responses (accuracy, RT). During the oddball task, participants responded to infrequent target stimuli (i.e., clip-art drawing of a cat) and were told not to respond to frequent nontarget stimuli (i.e., clip-art drawing of a dog) that were presented at a rate of 20% and 80%, respectively. Results indicated a positive relationship between fitness and cognitive function linked to the allocation of attentional resources to working memory in preadolescent children, as measured by the P3 potential. That is, higher-fit children evidenced larger P3 amplitude compared to the other three groups, which were not different from each other (Hillman, Castelli, & Buck, 2005).

Further, participants with greater aerobic fitness, regardless of age, evidenced faster P3 latency than sedentary participants, indicating that fitness was positively associated with cognitive processing speed (Hillman, Castelli, & Buck, 2005). Notably, fitness was also associated with task performance, as shorter RT was observed in higher-fit, compared to lower-fit, participants. Response accuracy was greater in higher-fit children relative to lower-fit children and also did not differ from either adult group. These findings indicate that aerobic fitness may be related to improvements in cognitive processes associated with attentional allocation during stimulus discrimination in preadolescent children, and provide a convincing argument for further investigation of underlying mechanisms that may be responsible for fitness effects on cognitive function in this population.

Although these data suggest a positive relationship between fitness and cognition, little research has addressed the relationship between fitness and executive control during cognitive development. According to Piaget, executive function begins to formulate around 8 to 9 months of age during the sensorimotor stage when goal-directed behavior becomes evident (Siegler, 1998). By the second year, children begin to grasp the concept of abstract rules. The comprehension of abstract rules allows for greater success on tests of working memory, processing speed, and interference control (Diamond, Towle, & Boyer, 1994). Early childhood (ages 3-7) is characterized by a marked improvement in certain executive control functions, such as inhibition and cognitive flexibility (Diamond, 2006), due to the development of the frontal lobes (e.g., Miyake et al., 2000; West, 1996). Executive control processes, including working memory, selective attention, and inhibitory control, improve throughout childhood and adolescence (Luciana & Nelson, 1998; Klenberg, Korkman, & Lahti-Nuuttila, 2001; Zelazo, Craik, & Booth, 2004), although performance relying on these processes remains poorer than that of young adults.

One task frequently used to study executive control is the Stroop Color-Word Task, which entails multiple cognitive processes including selective attention, response inhibition, interference control, and speeded responding (Adleman et al., 2002). The basic tenet underlying Stroop performance is that individuals must inhibit their prepotent response to read the words and activate a normally inhibited response to name the ink color in which the word is printed, thus resolving interference associated with reading the word (Adleman et al., 2002; Demetriou et al., 2002; MacLeod, 1991). Accordingly, participants read fewer words in the incongruent word-color condition due to response competition. In a study designed to gain understanding of the potential relationship between fitness and executive control, 74 preadolescent children between the ages of 7 and 12 years (37 boys; M = 9.4 years) completed a paper-and-pencil version of the Stroop Color-Word Task and completed the *Fitnessgram* (Buck, Hillman, & Castelli, 2008). During each of the three conditions of the Stroop task (word, color, color-word), participants were instructed to read aloud as many words as possible in 45 s. Results indicated that better performance on each of the three Stroop conditions was associated with age, IQ, and fitness. Specifically, older children and those with higher IQ read more words aloud correctly during each of the three conditions. Further, those children who completed more laps on the PACER test, indicating higher levels of aerobic fitness, correctly read more words during each condition.

These findings suggest that increased levels of fitness may benefit cognition during maturation and also that fitness may have a global relationship with cognition during this period of the life span. Interestingly, this contradicts previous literature with adult populations, which has indicated both a general and a selective relationship between fitness and cognition (Colcombe & Kramer, 2003; Kramer et al., 2005). That is, although research in adults has demonstrated general improvements in cognition with greater amounts of aerobic fitness, the relationship was disproportionately larger for tasks requiring extensive amounts of executive control (Colcombe & Kramer, 2003). However, the mechanisms underlying the relationship between aerobic fitness and improved cognitive performance remain poorly understood for both children and adults. In any case, these preliminary findings are encouraging and suggest that a more sensitive examination is warranted to achieve a better understanding of the relationship between fitness and cognition during different periods of the life span.

Accordingly, a second study from our laboratory examined neuroelectric concomitants of cognition in preadolescent children during performance of a task requiring variable amounts of executive control (Hillman et al., in press). Neuroelectric data were collected on 38 preadolescent children who were placed into higher (n = 19; 10 males) or lower (n = 19; 10 males) fitness groups based on aerobic capacity as measured by the PACER test of the *Fitnessgram* (Welk, Morris, & Falls, 2002). Participants completed congruent (i.e., HHHHH or SSSSS) and incongruent (i.e., HHSHH or SSHSS) conditions of the Eriksen flanker task (Eriksen & Eriksen, 1974), which required them to respond as quickly as possible to an array of letters presented on a computer monitor. Results indicated that P3 amplitude was larger over the parietal region of the scalp for higher- compared to lower-fit children across both conditions (Hillman et al., in press). Further, higher-fit children performed more accurately across conditions than lower-fit children, while group differences were not observed for RT latency. These findings indicate that fitness may be associated with better interference control in children and also—since they were obtained across conditions requiring variable amounts of interference control—that these cognitive benefits are nonselective during preadolescent childhood.

One translational ramification of the positive relationship between aerobic fitness and cognitive performance observed in the laboratory may relate to academic achievement testing, a common measure of cognitive performance in school-aged children. Castelli and colleagues (2007) investigated the relationship between different components of fitness (i.e., aerobic, muscle strength, flexibility) and academic achievement (Illinois State Achievement Test, ISAT) in 259 elementary school children in the 3rd and 5th grades (M = 9.5 years, female = 127). The *Fitnessgram* (Welk, Morris, & Falls, 2002) was administered to each student during regularly scheduled physical education classes. Children recruited for the study were representative of the population of the community along measures of race/ethnicity, socioeconomic status, and achievement test performance for the school district. The ISAT scores, administered each spring to children in 3rd through 8th grade, were collected with the *Fitnessgram* data. The ISAT tests grade-level student achievement in reading, writing, and mathematics for grades 3, 5, and 7 and science and social studies for grades 4, 6, and 8. Results indicated that only aerobic fitness was positively related to academic performance on mathematics and reading achievement, while body mass index was negatively related to scores on these achievement tests, independent of other variables (Castelli et al., 2007). Strength and flexibility fitness were not related to achievement test performance. These data provide preliminary evidence to suggest that higher aerobic fitness in school-age children may be associated with better academic performance, lend further support to the notion that fitness may be important to the development of cognitive health in this population, and provide additional evidence of a general relationship between fitness and cognition during development.

Potential Mechanisms for the Relationship Between Physical Activity and Neurocognitive Function

The underlying mechanisms by which physical activity affects cognitive function are not well understood. However, our understanding of the influences of physical activity on brain structure and function has significantly increased through human neuroimaging and animal model research. With regard to human neuroimaging research, the frontal regions of the brain have been heavily implicated in the modulation of top-down control on tasks requiring variable amounts of executive control. Specifically, disproportionate changes in brain structure with aging have been associated with age-related changes in executive control that are supported in large part by prefrontal and temporal regions of the brain (Robbins et al., 1998; Schretlen et al., 2000). Executive control function is inefficient and variable during the preadolescent years (Rueda et al., 2004) and has been related to immaturity of the frontal lobes during this period of the life span (Bunge et al., 2002). However, physical activity and aerobic exercise training have been related to changes in both structure and function of the prefrontal, frontal, and parietal cortices in older adults (Colcombe et al., 2004). Interestingly, selective improvements in executive control have been observed for aerobically trained adults, which may relate to changes in the health of these neural structures.

With regard to animal research, recent advancements have demonstrated several exercise-related changes at the molecular, vascular, and cellular levels of the brain. For example, aerobic exercise has been shown to increase neurochemicals such as brain-derived neurotrophin factor (BDNF; Neeper et al., 1995), insulin-like growth factor 1 (IGF1; Carro et al., 2001), serotonin (Blomstrand et al., 1989), and dopamine (Spirduso & Farrar, 1981), which have been found to improve plasticity and neuronal survival and underlie learning and memory in adult rats (Cotman & Berchtold, 2002) and neonatal rat pups (Parnpiansil et al., 2003). Other animal research has evidenced the development of new capillaries in the cerebellum with aerobic exercise, presumably to support increased neuronal firing, in rodents (Black et al., 1990; Isaacs et al., 1992) and primates (Rhyu et al., 2003). Importantly, these exercise-induced changes in neural structures have been linked to greater resting blood flow and an increased ability to respond to greater oxygen demands in comparison to values in sedentary controls (Swain et al., 2003).

The relationship between physical activity–induced changes in the basic neurobiology and neuroelectric (i.e., ERP) correlates of human cognition is tenuous. However, several brain structures (i.e., prefrontal, frontal, temporal, parietal) and neurochemicals (i.e., dopamine) most influenced by physical activity have also been related to the modulation of ERP components. The precise neural tissue mediating the P3 response is unknown, since this ERP component likely reflects a network of neural circuitry and generators. However, discrimination tasks requiring attentional focus are thought to elicit frontal lobe activation (Posner, 1992; Posner & Petersen, 1990), with ERP (i.e., P3a) and fMRI studies demonstrating greater frontal lobe activity in response to rare or alerting stimuli (Polich, 2004). The ACC is activated when working memory representations of the stimulus environment change, which in turn signals the inferotemporal lobe for stimulus maintenance (i.e., memory storage). The P3 (i.e., P3b) component is elicited when attentional resources are allocated for subsequent memory updating after stimulus evaluation (Polich, 2004). It is hypothesized that this occurs when memory storage operations initiated in the hippocampal formation are transmitted to the parietal cortex, which is typically where the P3 exhibits maximal amplitude in the scalp distribution (Squire & Kandell, 1999; Knight, 1996). Thus, the neuroelectric events that underlie P3 generation occur from the interaction between frontal lobe and hippocampal/ temporal-parietal function (Knight, 1996; Polich, 2004) to modulate attentional control over the contents of working memory (Polich, 2004).

More is known about the neural circuitry underlying the response-locked ERN and Pe components. As discussed previously, the source of the ERN has been localized to the dorsal ACC, and the source of the Pe has been localized to the rostral ACC using several imaging measures. The Pe and P3 components are strongly correlated and are thought to reflect similar attentional processes (Davies et al., 2001). Gehring and Knight (2000) have also observed that the ACC exhibits a functional interaction with the prefrontal cortex during action monitoring processes. In addition, Holroyd and Coles' (2002) reinforcement learning model suggests that the ERN is modulated through a reduction in dopaminergic activity that disinhibits the ACC. Given the early developmental and age-related changes in the structure and function of the frontal lobe, changes in dopamine levels (Brozoski et al., 1979) during preadolescence and older adulthood, and the functional interaction between the ACC and prefrontal cortex, processes subserved by these brain regions may be especially amenable to intervention during these periods of the life span. Interestingly, researchers have suggested that aerobic exercise affects both activation of the ACC (Colcombe et al., 2004) and dopaminergic activity (Wang et al., 2000), indicating that aerobic exercise training may be one such intervention leading to improvements in cognitive performance—which can easily be monitored through the modulation of various ERP components.

Future Directions

Despite the growing body of literature on the relationship between physical activity and neuroelectric indices of cognition that has emerged in recent years, there is a need to gain a better understanding of this relationship. Specifically, since physical activity participation has been found to benefit cognitive function during earlier periods of the human life span, most notably during preadolescent development, future research efforts must focus on how early in the life span these differences emerge. Further, from a life span perspective, it is important to determine the time course of this relationship, as there appears to be a shift during maturation in which physical activity effects change from global to selective aspects of cognition. That is, research with adult populations clearly indicates that physical activity effects on cognition are disproportionately larger for executive control tasks, whereas in children the data indicate a more global relationship across tasks and task types. A better understanding of this relationship may also provide information to cognitive neuroscientists about important developmental changes in brain structure and function that coincide with the development of higher-level cognitive functioning, such as executive control.

Several other important aspects of this relationship have not been thoroughly investigated. For example, the amount, intensity, and duration of physical activity necessary to provide positive changes in cognitive function are as yet unknown. Given that the various cognitive functions are mediated by different brain structures, it is obvious that this relationship is not straightforward. Since executive control deteriorates more extensively than other types of cognition, determining the amount, intensity, and duration of physical activity needed to improve this aspect of cognition is of the utmost importance. However, executive control in and of itself is not unitary, and thus determining this relationship within the subset of processes that comprise executive control will prove challenging. Future examinations of this topic will also have to involve more rigorous scientific methods than those reviewed in this chapter. That is, the vast majority of research to date has utilized cross-sectional designs involving groups that fall along the extremes of the physical activity or aerobic fitness continuum. Further efforts will need to employ randomized controlled designs so that causality in this relationship can be better inferred.

Finally, little is known about the majority of neuroelectric processes that occur during information processing. Most research thus far has focused on the P3 component, while a subset of studies have focused on various other ERP components. Hence, although our understanding of processes subsumed by the P3 is reasonable, little is known about other cognitive processes involved in the stimulus–response relationship. Future efforts clearly need to address this paucity in the literature to determine whether certain processes are disproportionately influenced by physical activity relative to others. Despite the need for these future research efforts, the knowledge base on physical activity and neuroelectric indices of cognition has experienced substantial growth during the last decade. These efforts have led to a deeper understanding of lifestyle factors that promote better cognitive health and function across the life span.

CHAPTER 7

Effects of Acute Exercise on Event-Related Brain Potentials

Keita Kamijo, PhD

Cognition and Action Research Group,
Institute for Human Science and Biomedical Engineering,
National Institute of Advanced Industrial Science and Technology (AIST)

Over the past several decades there has been increased interest in the influence of physical activity, and in particular aerobic exercise, on human cognitive processing. Most studies of the effect of exercise on cognitive processing have examined behavioral indices of task performance, such as reaction time (RT) and response accuracy (see Tomporowski & Ellis, 1986; Tomporowski, 2003 for review). However, in recent years, our understanding of the relationship between exercise and cognitive processing has progressed beyond the study of behavioral responses to include the study of neuroelectric correlates of behavior. The work in our laboratory has focused on examination of the effects of exercise and physical activity on event-related brain potentials (ERPs).

Event-related brain potentials are a basic, noninvasive method for investigating the electrical system of the brain. They have been used to assess aspects of human information processing (Hruby & Marsalek, 2003), and provide insight into some of the underlying mechanisms involved in cognitive functioning. Recent studies investigating the effects of both acute and chronic exercise on ERPs have shown evidence for changes in cognitive processing following exercise (see Kramer & Hillman, 2006 for review). This chapter focuses on the impact of acute exercise on ERPs.

Most studies investigating the effects of acute exercise on ERPs have focused on the P3 component (Duzova et al., 2005; Grego et al., 2004; Hillman, Snook, & Jerome, 2003; Kamijo et al., 2004b; Magnié et al., 2000; Nakamura et al., 1999; Pontifex & Hillman, 2007; Yagi, Coburn, Estes, & Arruda, 1999). The P3 is an endogenous component of the stimulus-locked ERP that is believed to provide an index of the brain activity required for the maintenance of working memory when a mental model of the stimulus environment is updated (Donchin & Coles, 1988). The amplitude of the P3 component is thought to be proportional to the amount of attentional resources devoted to a given stimulus or task (Kida et al., 2004; Schubert et al., 1998); the latency is considered to measure stimulus classification speed or stimulus evaluation time and is generally unrelated to response selection processes (McCarthy & Donchin, 1981; Pfefferbaum et al., 1983).

The studies on the effects of acute exercise have indicated that P3 changes are observed both during and following acute exercise. However, the experimental literature is replete with contradictory findings, which have led several authors to identify the following methodological factors that need to be carefully controlled in acute exercise ERP studies: (1) the physical fitness of participants, (2) the intensity and duration of physical exercise, (3) the nature of the psychological task, and (4) the time at which the psychological task is administered relative to the acute exercise bout (Collardeau et al., 2001).

The purpose of this chapter is to provide an overview of the relationship between acute exercise and ERPs, whenever possible giving attention to the methodological constraints suggested by Collardeau and colleagues. The first section of the chapter focuses on methodological differences across acute exercise studies that have measured the P3 wave. The second section deals with other ERP components, such as the earlier stimulus-locked components (e.g., N1, P2, and N2), the contingent negative variation (CNV), and the error-related negativity (ERN). The chapter concludes with some speculation about the effects of acute exercise on ERP indices of cognitive processing in older adults.

Acute Exercise and the P3

Table 7.1 summarizes the acute exercise studies that have measured the P3 component. As can be seen, the findings across the various studies are inconsistent. In a discussion of the extant literature it is necessary to consider a number of factors, including differences in the physical fitness of the study participants; differences in the intensity, mode, and duration of the exercise intervention; differences in the nature of psychological tasks employed and the cognitive processes that are tapped by such tasks; and finally, differences in the timing with regard to when the P3 was measured relative to the acute exercise bout. When these differences are taken into consideration, it is not surprising that there is little consensus about the effect of acute aerobic exercise on P3. Each of these methodological differences is considered later.

Physical Fitness of Participants

On the surface, it would appear that the majority of research in this area has used similar subject samples, since most have examined young adults. However, further consideration shows that the samples differ in several important ways. That is, several studies have used regularly active individuals or athletes (Grego et al., 2004; Hillman et al., 2003; Nakamura et

Table 7.1 Methodological Differences in P3 Studies

No.	Investigators	Participants	Exercise	Psychological task	Timing of P3 measurement
1	Duzova et al. (2005)	31 male soccer players (high physically active, 11; medium, 10; low, 10) Age: 18-26 years $\dot{V}O_2$max: not indicated	Anaerobic loading coordination test Intensity: maximal exercise (about 190 bpm) Duration: 45 s	Auditory oddball task (count)	Before exercise, also after participants' body temperature and HR returned to baseline level
2	Grego et al. (2004)	12 male cyclists Age: 29 years $\dot{V}O_2$max: 69 ml · kg^{-1} · min^{-1}	Cycling exercise Intensity: 66% $\dot{V}O_2$max Duration: 180 min	Auditory oddball task (count)	Before, during (3, 36, 72, 108, 144 min), immediately after, and 15 min after exercise
3	Hillman et al. (2003)*	10 males, 9 females (participated in regular physical activity) Age: 20.5 years $\dot{V}O_2$max: 48.4 ml · kg^{-1} · min^{-1}	Treadmill exercise Intensity: 162.4 bpm (83.5% HRmax) Duration: 30 min	Eriksen flanker task	After participants' HR returned to within 10% of baseline level: mean = 48 min after exercise
4	Kamijo et al. (2004)*	12 males Age: 24.9 years $\dot{V}O_2$max: not indicated	Cycling exercise Intensity: until volitional exhaustion (high: 190.2 bpm at the final stage of GXT), RPE 12-14 (medium: 118.2 bpm), RPE 7-9 (low: 84.4 bpm) Duration: 18 min	Go/NoGo RT task	Immediately (less than 3 min) after exercise

(continued)

Table 7.1 *(continued)*

No.	Investigators	Participants	Exercise	Psychological task	Timing of P3 measurement
5	Magnié et al. (2000) *	20 males (10 cyclists, 10 sedentary) Age: 21.2 (cyclists), 22.9 (sedentary) years $\dot{V}O_2$max: cyclists, 63.8; sedentary, 47.4 ml · kg^{-1} · min^{-1}	Cycling exercise Intensity: until volitional exhaustion Duration: not indicated	Auditory oddball task (count)	Before exercise and after participants' body temperature and HR returned to baseline level: mean = 69 (cyclists), 52 (sedentary) min after exercise
6	Nakamura et al. (1999)	7 male joggers Age: 34.6 years $\dot{V}O_2$max: not indicated	Jogging Intensity: comfortable and self-paced cadence Duration: 30 min	Auditory oddball task (count)	Before and 10 min after exercise
7	Pontifex & Hillman (2007)	15 males, 26 females Age: 20.2 years $\dot{V}O_2$max: 38.3 ml · kg^{-1} · min^{-1}	Cycling exercise Intensity: 60% HRmax Duration: 6 min	Modified flanker task that incorporated arrays of arrows	Before (half the participants) and during exercise, and after participants' HR returned to baseline level: mean = 6.3 min after exercise (other half)
8	Yagi et al. (1999)	12 males, 12 females Age: 19.9 (males), 20.6 (females) years $\dot{V}O_2$max: not indicated	Cycling exercise Intensity: 130-150 bpm Duration: 10 min	Both auditory and visual oddball task	Before, during, and immediately after exercise

*Hillman et al. (2003) and Kamijo et al. (2004b) recorded baseline ERPs on a different day from the exercise session.

Note: Ages listed are average age of study parcipants. HR = heart rate, RPE = rating of perceived exertion, and RT = reaction time.

al., 1999), while others have used untrained or nonathlete populations (Kamijo et al., 2004b; Pontifex & Hillman, 2007; Yagi et al., 1999). The studies that recorded P3 in athletes and active subjects following exercise showed greater allocation of attentional resources or faster cognitive processing speed (larger P3 amplitude and faster latency, respectively; Hillman et al., 2003; Nakamura et al., 1999), or both. Kamijo and colleagues (2004b) also observed larger P3 amplitudes after moderate-intensity exercise in nonathletes. These findings suggest that after moderate-intensity exercise, similar neuroelectric responses are observed across fitness levels in young adults.

On the other hand, several studies that recorded ERPs during exercise showed lower response accuracy or longer P3 latency (or both) regardless of the participants' physical fitness (Grego et al., 2004; Pontifex & Hillman, 2007; Yagi et al., 1999). For example, Grego and colleagues (2004) examined the neuroelectric responses of trained cyclists during long-duration cycling at approximately 66% of $\dot{V}O_2$max. The P3 component was measured at regular intervals during 180 min of cycling exercise (i.e., 3, 36, 72, 108, and 144 min). P3 amplitude was found to increase significantly between the 72nd and 108th min, whereas P3 latency was significantly longer between the 108th and 144th min (see figure 7.1). These findings suggest an increase in the allocation of attentional resources but slower cognitive processing speed during prolonged aerobic exercise (Grego et al., 2004).

Pontifex and Hillman (2007) examined the effects of in-task, short-duration (6 min), moderate-intensity (60% HRmax) cycling exercise on neuroelectric response of young adults ($\dot{V}O_2$max: 38.3 ml $\cdot$ kg^{-1} $\cdot$ min^{-1}). Larger P3 amplitudes and longer P3 latencies were observed during exercise relative to rest. These findings suggest that the addition of exercise during performance of a cognitive task creates a dual-task environment in which the participant must successfully negotiate the demands imposed by the cognitive task and allocate resources toward the maintenance of steady-state exercise (Pontifex & Hillman, 2007). It was further proposed that inefficiency of neural resource allocation occurred during the moderate-intensity cycling exercise condition for untrained nonexpert cyclists. In contrast, inefficiency of neuroelectric resources during cycling exercise has not been shown during the early phases of exercise for experienced cyclists, probably because cyclists are more familiar with cycling exercise. However, inefficiency of cognitive functioning might appear even for trained cyclists during prolonged exercise (longer than 1 hr) when central and peripheral fatigue occur.

Magnié and colleagues (2000) examined individuals with higher and lower levels of aerobic fitness to determine whether differences in P3 could be found following an acute bout of maximal cycling exercise. Trained cyclists ($\dot{V}O_2$max: 63.8 ml $\cdot$ kg^{-1} $\cdot$ min^{-1}) and sedentary participants ($\dot{V}O_2$max: 47.4 ml $\cdot$ kg^{-1} $\cdot$ min^{-1}) were compared to determine the relationship of

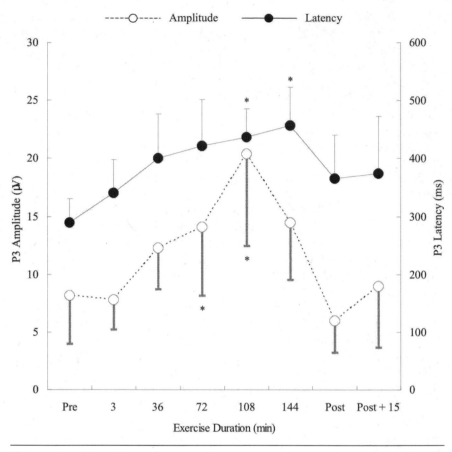

Figure 7.1 Mean P3 amplitude and latency in 180 min cycling exercise. Significantly different from the 3rd min, *$p < 0.05$.

Reprinted from *Neuroscience Letters*, vol 364, F. Grego, J.M. Vallier, M. Collardeau, S. Berman, P. Ferrari, M. Candito, P. Bayer, M.N. Magnié, and J. Brisswalter, "Effects of long duration exercise on cognitive function, blood glucose, and counterregulatory hormones in male cyclists," pgs. 76-80, Copyright 2004, with permission from Elsevier.

aerobic fitness to neuroelectric responses to an acute bout of exercise. Postexercise ERPs were measured immediately after body temperature and heart rate (HR) returned to preexercise levels in an attempt to account for the influence of general physiological arousal associated with intense exercise. Larger P3 amplitudes and shorter P3 latencies were observed following the bout of maximal exercise in all participants regardless of fitness level. This finding suggests that aerobic fitness levels do not influence cognitive function associated with acute aerobic exercise.

Duzova and colleagues (2005) divided soccer players into three physical activity groups (high active: >5 hr/week of training, moderate active: 2 to 5 hr/week of training, low active: <2 hr/week of training) and investigated the effects on ERPs of a maximal anaerobic coordination exercise with a duration of about 45 s (HR during the task was about 190 bpm). Their findings also showed no significant differences in P3 amplitude or latency among the activity groups. Furthermore, the P3 component was unchanged by the exercise intervention, with no differences observed between pre- and postexercise. Collectively, the data from these two studies indicate that the aerobic fitness of individuals is not related to the modulation of the P3 following acute exercise. This is of interest because long-term aerobic exercise and aerobic fitness have consistently been found to influence the P3.

Other research on changes in performance as a function of acute exercise has suggested that acute exercise effects on cognitive function can be influenced by the aerobic fitness of the participants (Gutin & DiGennaro, 1968a, 1968b; Sjoberg, 1980). However, not all studies have shown such a relationship (Tomporowski, Ellis, & Stephens, 1987; Travlos & Marisi, 1995). The former studies cited suggested that participants with greater fitness are better able to withstand the detrimental effects of physical stress than are less fit individuals (Gutin & DiGennaro, 1968a, 1968b; Sjoberg, 1980). To our knowledge, only two studies have addressed interactive effects of acute exercise and physical fitness on P3 (Magnié et al., 2000; Duzova et al., 2005), and additional research on these issues is needed.

Exercise Intensity and Duration

Studies have shown large differences with respect to the type of acute exercise interventions employed. With regard to exercise intensity, P3 studies are divided in two groups: those that have employed moderate-intensity (Grego et al., 2004; Nakamura et al., 1999; Pontifex & Hillman, 2007; Yagi et al., 1999) and high-intensity (Duzova et al., 2005; Hillman et al., 2003; Magnié et al., 2000) exercise. From the standpoint of exercise duration, most studies have used about 20 to 30 min exercise bouts (Hillman et al., 2003; Kamijo et al. 2004b; Magnié et al., 2000; Nakamura et al., 1999), with a few exceptions (e.g., Duzova et al., 2005: 45 s; Grego et al., 2004: 180 min). Additionally, two ERP studies have used relatively short bouts and measured cognitive function during exercise (Pontifex & Hillman, 2007: 6 min; Yagi et al., 1999: 10 min).

Kamijo and colleagues (2004b) investigated the influence of exercise intensity on cognitive processing using the P3. The P3 component was recorded during a nonexercise baseline session and again immediately after low-intensity (rating of perceived exertion: RPE 7-9), medium-intensity (RPE: 12-14), and high-intensity (until volitional exhaustion) cycling exercise to determine the differential influence of various exercise intensities on cognition. Compared to baseline values, P3 amplitude decreased after high-intensity exercise and increased after medium-intensity exercise, and there was no change after low-intensity exercise (figure 7.2). The findings

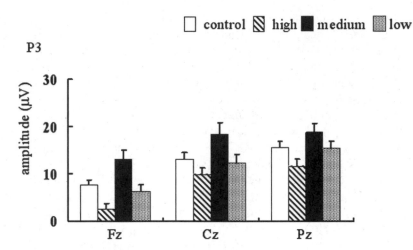

P3

NoGo P3

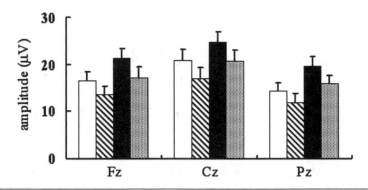

Figure 7.2 Mean P3 (upper) and NoGo P3 (lower) amplitudes from the Fz, Cz, and Pz electrode sites in a nonexercise control condition and after high-, medium-, and low-intensity exercise.

With kind permission from Springer Science & Business Media: *Europrean Journal of Applied Physiology*, "Differential influences of exercise intensity on information processing in the central nervous system," 92, 2004, pgs. 305-311, K. Kamijo, Y. Nishihira, A. Hatta, T. Kaneda, T. Wasaka, T. Kida, and K. Kuroiwa.

suggest that changes in P3 amplitude may be described by an inverted-U distribution with respect to exercise intensity. In other words, P3 indices of cognition may be facilitated immediately after moderate-intensity exercise and degraded after high-intensity exercise. The findings support the results of Nakamura and colleagues (1999), which indicated that moderate-intensity exercise facilitates cognitive processing.

Other research employing high-intensity exercise, such as that of Hillman and colleagues (2003) and Magnié and colleagues (2000), recorded the P3 only after participants' body temperature and HR returned to baseline level (about 50-70 min after exercise). These studies showed larger amplitudes or shorter latencies (or both) following relatively high-intensity acute exercise compared to baseline. These findings suggest that cognitive processing as reflected by the P3 component deteriorates immediately after high-intensity exercise but returns to baseline or is enhanced after recovery. It has been speculated that P3 changes following acute exercise might be influenced by catecholamine activity. That is, the plasma concentration of catecholamines increases linearly with exercise intensity and duration and then decreases gradually after exercise (e.g., Kjaer, 1989; Kjaer, Farrell, Christensen, & Galbo, 1986). It has also been suggested that plasma catecholamines are related to cognitive performance (Chmura et al., 1998; Chmura, Nazar, & Kaciuba-Uscilko, 1994; McMorris & Graydon, 2000). Chmura and colleagues (1994) investigated the relationship between plasma catecholamines and cognitive performance in a graded exercise test and suggested that a relationship between response speed and plasma catecholamines may be described by a U-shaped distribution.

With regard to exercise duration, Grego and colleagues (2004) observed no changes in P3 amplitude following a long duration of exercise (180 min) at a moderate intensity. This suggests that moderate-intensity exercise facilitates cognitive function up to a certain point in time but that long duration may negate these beneficial effects due to central or peripheral fatigue or both. In addition, Duzova and colleagues (2005) indicated that the P3 component was unchanged following maximal and very short-duration (45 s) anaerobic exercise. This finding suggests that P3 is unchanged following high-intensity exercise when the exercise duration is very short.

Tomporowski and Ellis (1986) provide some basis from which to interpret the inconsistent findings described here, suggesting that exercise may initially facilitate cognitive processing by directly affecting the central nervous system but that as exercise intensity or duration increases, the facilitative effects of the activity may be negated by the debilitating effects of muscular fatigue. Accordingly, differences in exercise intensity and duration would affect cognitive processing due to their differential effects on fatigue. Additional research is needed to more carefully examine how exercise intensity and duration influence cognition.

Nature of the Psychological Task

Traditionally, the P3 has been evoked using a simple stimulus discrimination task known as the oddball paradigm. The vast majority of P3 studies investigating the effects of acute exercise have used this paradigm (Grego et al., 2004; Magnié et al., 2000; Nakamura et al., 1999; Yagi et al., 1999), in which a frequent (standard) stimulus and an infrequent (target) stimulus are presented, the latter occurring on approximately 20% of the trials.

The participants are required to react to the presence of the target stimulus with a motor response, typically a button press, or by silently counting the number of target stimuli. The response accuracy of this task is high, so the task is considered relatively simple.

Chodzko-Zajko (1991) suggested that effortful or attentionally demanding tasks may be more sensitive to the beneficial effects of exercise than tasks that require minimal effort. That is, the effects of acute exercise on cognitive processing differ depending on the nature of the psychological task. Hillman and colleagues (2003) focused on this issue using a modified flanker task that manipulates executive control requirements. Perner and Lang (1999) defined executive control as "processes responsible for the higher-level control necessary for maintaining a specified goal and for selecting it when faced with distracting alternatives" (p. 337). The prefrontal cortex has been considered an important structure for executive control (see Funahashi, 2001 for review). It includes functions important for the organization of action, mental flexibility, complex discrimination, error monitoring, response selection, and response inhibition (Meyer & Kieras, 1997; Norman & Shallice, 1986). One paradigm that has been shown to effectively manipulate executive control requirements is the Eriksen flanker task (Eriksen & Eriksen, 1974). This task consists of two types of stimuli whose central target letter is flanked with noise letters (e.g., HHHHH for congruent stimulus, SSHSS for incongruent stimulus). Congruent stimuli elicit faster and more accurate responses, and incongruent stimuli cause decreased response speed and accuracy (Eriksen & Schultz, 1979). The latter require greater amounts of executive control since incongruent arrays result in response delay due to activation of an incorrect response before evaluation is completed (Kramer et al., 1994; Kramer & Jacobson, 1991). Hillman and colleagues (2003) suggested that acute exercise might have a larger effect on task components requiring extensive amounts of executive control, relative to task components with smaller executive control requirements, since they observed shorter P3 latencies only for the incongruent trials (figure 7.3). Kamijo and colleagues (2004b) also indicated that "NoGo" P3, interpreted as a reflection of inhibitory process (i.e., a different aspect of executive control; Bokura, Yamaguchi, & Kobayashi, 2001; Bruin, Wijers, & van Staveren, 2001; Falkenstein, Hoormann, & Hohnsbein, 1999; Fallgatter & Strik, 1999), changed after cycling exercise. Together, these two studies suggest that various aspects of executive control may be especially sensitive to the effects of acute exercise.

Further, Pontifex and Hillman (2007) investigated the effects of in-task, moderate-intensity aerobic exercise on neuroelectric and behavioral indices of interference control using the flanker task. Results indicated that in-task exercise was related to poorer response accuracy only for incongruent trials relative to rest, and larger P3 amplitude and longer latency were observed during exercise relative to rest for both incongruent and congruent trials.

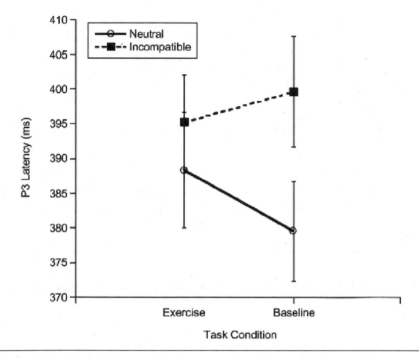

Figure 7.3 Mean P3 latency for the neutral and incompatible conditions of the Eriksen flanker task during exercise and baseline sessions.

Adapted from *International Journal of Psychophysiology,* vol 48, C.H. Hillman, E.M. Snook, and G.J. Jerome, "Acute cardiovascular exercise and executive control function," pgs. 307-314, Copyright 2003, with permission from Elsevier.

These findings suggest that acute exercise influences executive control function. Further, because P3 varies as a function of the degree of executive control required by a task, this may be a sensitive measure for assessing cognitive responses to acute exercise stress.

Although these data suggest that acute exercise influences cognitive performance, a number of issues still need to be resolved regarding the specific nature of the psychological task. For example, although Hillman and colleagues (2003) indicated that acute exercise affects the neuroelectric processes underlying executive control, only mixed support has been found for the hypothesis that general arousal is responsible for exercise-induced effects on P3. Specifically, P3 latency for trials requiring minimal effort did not show this effect, as longer latencies were observed following exercise (figure 7.3). Thus, additional research is needed on the relationship between acute exercise and the nature of the psychological task using tasks that manipulate executive control requirements.

Timing of P3 Measurement

From the perspective of the timing of P3 measurements, studies have been classified into three main categories according to whether measurements are taken during exercise (Grego et al., 2004; Pontifex & Hillman, 2007; Yagi et al., 1999), immediately after exercise (Grego et al., 2004; Kamijo et al., 2004b; Nakamura et al., 1999; Yagi et al., 1999), or after the participants' body temperature, HR, or both return to baseline levels (Duzova et al., 2005; Hillman et al., 2003; Magnié et al., 2000).

In the studies measuring P3 during exercise, larger P3 amplitudes and longer P3 latencies have been observed during exercise relative to rest, suggesting inefficiency of neural resource allocation during exercise (Grego et al., 2004; Pontifex & Hillman, 2007). However, Yagi and colleagues (1999) observed shorter RT, lower response accuracy, smaller P3 amplitude, and shorter P3 latency during exercise, suggesting a reduction in the allocation of available attentional resources but faster cognitive processing speed during exercise relative to rest. Yet a speed–accuracy trade-off was evident given the increased number of errors that accompanied the faster responding.

With respect to studies measuring P3 after exercise, the findings are also inconsistent. Kamijo and colleagues (2004b) observed smaller P3 amplitude immediately after high-intensity exercise, whereas Hillman and colleagues (2003) and Magnié and colleagues (2000) found larger P3 amplitude or shorter P3 latency (or both) after participants' HR or body temperature returned to baseline levels following relatively high-intensity acute exercise (about 50-70 min after exercise). The data from the latter studies are interesting because they suggest that body temperature and HR influence P3 latency (Geisler & Polich, 1990). However, others suggest that increases in body temperature due to acute exercise result in decreased arousal level both during and following exercise (Nielsen et al., 2001), and that P3 may be influenced by changes in arousal level (Polich & Kok, 1995). Therefore, in ERP studies on effects of acute exercise, it is recommended that ERP recording be performed before exercise, immediately after exercise, and after body temperature, HR, or both return to preexercise level.

With respect to the recording of baseline data, studies can be broken down into two groups. Most studies use a pre–post study design (Duzova et al., 2005; Grego et al., 2004; Magnié et al., 2000; Nakamura et al., 1999; Yagi et al., 1999). However, P3 amplitudes decline or habituate after repeated stimulus presentation because the updating of the neural model of the stimulus environment becomes automated (e.g., Ravden & Polich, 1998; Lew & Polich, 1993). Thus, P3 may be influenced by not only acute exercise but also the habituation or general practice effect in pre–post studies. On the other hand, Hillman and colleagues (2003) and Kamijo and colleagues (2004b) recorded the baseline session at the same time but on a different day from the exercise session and counterbalanced the study sessions to eliminate the habituation effect. It is recommended that the baseline session be conducted at the same time on a different day from the exercise session in ERP studies investigating effects of acute exercise.

In conclusion, there is evidence to suggest that P3 changes are observed following high-intensity exercise even after body temperature, HR, or both have returned to preexercise levels (Hillman et al., 2003; Magnié et al., 2000). However, there is a paucity of data regarding how long the effects of acute exercise on cognitive processing continue. Although it is speculated that these changes depend on exercise intensity, duration, and physical fitness of the participants, additional studies that include serial assessment of behavioral measures and ERPs after acute exercise are needed.

Acute Exercise and Other ERP Components

Event-related potential waveforms contain components that span a continuum between the exogenous potentials (obligatory responses determined by the physical characteristics of the eliciting event) and the endogenous potentials (manifestations of information processing in the brain that may or may not be invoked by the eliciting event; Picton et al., 2000). Event-related potentials are associated with sensory, cognitive, or motor events and can be elicited by either a stimulus or a response. Because the temporal resolution of these measurements is rapid, ERPs can accurately measure the time at which processing activities take place in the human brain (Picton et al., 2000). That is, the ERP waveforms provide information regarding the temporal aspects of information processing.

Table 7.2 summarizes acute exercise studies that measured ERP components other than the P3. This section provides a summary of the research findings from these studies.

VEPs and BAEPs

Several studies have investigated the effects of acute exercise on visual or auditory pathways (or both) using visual evoked potentials (VEPs), brainstem auditory evoked potentials (BAEPs), or both (Magnié et al., 1998; Ozmerdivenli et al., 2005; Thomas, Jones, Scott, & Rosenberg, 1991). Visual evoked potentials are used to assess the central visual pathway and provide an objective assessment of human visual functioning (see Walsh, Kane, & Butler, 2005 for review). Those evoked by pattern-reversal stimuli include a triphasic waveform: N75, P100, and N145. On the other hand, BAEPs include a sequence of five peaks (I-V). The usefulness of BAEPs can be extended by knowledge of the central auditory structures from which the different waveform components of BAEP originate (Biacabe, Chevallier, Avan, & Bonfils, 2001).

Table 7.2   Detailed Outline of Other ERP Studies

No.	Investigators	Participants	Exercise	Component (psychological task)	Timing of P3 measurement
1	Duzova et al. (2005)	31 male soccer players (high physically active, 11; medium, 10; low, 10) Age: 18-26 years $\dot{V}O_2$max: not indicated	Anaerobic loading coordination test Intensity: maximal exercise (about 190 bpm) Duration: 45 s	N2 (auditory odd-ball task; count)	Before exercise, also after participants' body temperature and HR returned to baseline level
2	Kamijo et al. (2004a)*	12 males Age: 24.9 years $\dot{V}O_2$max: not indicated	Cycling exercise Intensity: until volitional exhaustion (high: 190.2 bpm at the final stage of GXT), RPE 12-14 (medium: 118.2 bpm), RPE 7-9 (low: 84.4 bpm) Duration: 18 min	CNV (Go/NoGo RT task)	Immediately (less than 3 min) after exercise
3	Magnié et al. (1998)	16 males (8 cyclists, 8 sedentary) Age: 20.9 (cyclists), 23.5 (sedentary) years $\dot{V}O_2$max: cyclists, 64.4; sedentary, 46.4 ml · kg^{-1} · min^{-1}	Cycling exercise Intensity: until volitional exhaustion Duration: not indicated	VEP (checkerboard pattern reversal) BAEP (click)	Before exercise and after participants' body temperature returned to baseline level: mean = 54 (cyclists), 72 (sedentary) min after exercise

4	Magnié et al. (2000)	20 males (10 cyclists, 10 sedentary) Age: 21.2 (cyclists), 22.9 (sedentary) years $\dot{V}O_2$max: cyclists, 63.8; sedentary, 47.4 ml · kg⁻¹ · min⁻¹	Cycling exercise Intensity: until volitional exhaustion Duration: not indicated	N1, P2, N2 (auditory oddball task; count) N400 (semantic incongruity task)	Before exercise and after participants' body temperature and HR returned to baseline level: mean = 69 (cyclists), 52 (sedentary) min after exercise
5	Nakamura et al. (1999)	7 male joggers Age: 34.6 years $\dot{V}O_2$max: not indicated	Jogging Intensity: comfortable and self-paced cadence Duration: 30 min	N1 (auditory oddball task; count)	Before and 10 min after exercise
6	Ozmerdivenli et al. 2005	16 males, 16 females (9 volleyball players, 7 sedentary, for each gender) Age: 20.2 (mv), 19.6 (ms), 21.1 (fv), 21.4 (fs) years $\dot{V}O_2$max: 51.3, 44.2, 38.8, 30.4 ml · kg⁻¹ · min⁻¹	Treadmill exercise Intensity: 60-70% HRmax Duration: 30 min	VEP (checkerboard pattern reversal)	Before exercise and after participants' body temperature returned to baseline level
7	Pontifex and Hillman (2007)	15 males, 26 females Age: 20.2 years $\dot{V}O_2$max: 38.3 ml · kg⁻¹ · min⁻¹	Cycling exercise Intensity: 60% HRmax Duration: 6 min	N1, P2, N2 (modified flanker task)	Before (half the participants) and during exercise, and after participants' HR returned to baseline level: mean = 6.3 min after exercise (other half)

(continued)

Table 7.2 *(continued)*

No.	Investigators	Participants	Exercise	Component (psychological task)	Timing of P3 measurement
8	Themanson and Hillman (2006)*	14 males, 14 males (7 higher fit, 7 lower fit, for each gender) Age: 20.1 (higher fit), 20.6 (lower fit) years $\dot{V}O_2$max: higher fit, 56.3; lower fit, 38.7 ml · kg^{-1} · min^{-1}	Treadmill exercise Intensity: 161.0 bpm (82.8% HRmax) Duration: 30 min	ERN, Pe, N2 (Eriksen flanker task)	After participants' HR returned to within 10% of baseline level: mean = 40 min after exercise
9	Thomas et al. (1991)	8 males, 8 females Age: 21-23 years $\dot{V}O_2$max: not indicated	Cycling exercise Intensity: moderate for the given participant (100-200 W) Duration: 20 min	BAEP (tone pip)	Before and immediately after exercise, and 15 min after the last recording

Note: Kamijo et al. (2004a) and Themanson & Hillman (2006) recorded baseline ERPs on a different day from the exercise session. CNV = contingent negative variation, RT = reaction time, HR = heart rate, GXT = graded exercise test, RPE = rating of perceived exertion, VEP = visual evoked potential, ERN = error-related negativity, Pe = error positivity, BAEP = brainstem auditory evoked potential.

Magnié and colleagues (1998) investigated the effects of maximal cycling exercise on VEPs and BAEPs. They recorded VEPs and BAEPs after participants' body temperature returned to baseline levels (about 55-70 min after exercise). They found that the VEP and BAEP waves did not change when body temperature returned to preexercise level. In contrast, Thomas and colleagues (1991) recorded BAEPs immediately after moderate cycling exercise and found that the latencies of waves III and V were significantly shorter with higher body temperature than before exercise. Thomas and colleagues suggested that elevation of body temperature by acute exercise shortens the latency of the evoked potentials. However, Ozmerdivenli and colleagues (2005) found that N145 latencies of VEPs after treadmill exercise (60-70% HRmax) in inactive female participants were longer after than before exercise, although the VEPs were recorded after body temperature recovery to preexercise level.

N1, P2, and N2

Occurring after the VEPs or BAEPs are several later peaks including N1, P2, N2, P3, and N400, which reflect more integrative cognitive processing. In some studies, the effects of acute exercise on earlier ERP components (i.e., N1, P2, and N2), collected during an oddball task or other choice RT tasks, have been evaluated. In general, N1, P2, and N2 are elicited before the appearance of the P3 component. The N1 component is believed to reflect the operation of a discrimination process within the focus of attention (Vogel & Luck, 2000), and it is speculated that the P2 component is an indicator of the stimulus classification process (Crowley & Colrain, 2004). Although it is clear that N1 peak is dependent on stimulus modality, the topography of P2 appears to be similar across auditory, visual, and somatosensory modalities (see Crowley & Colrain, 2004 for review). It is thought that the P2 may have two or more different sources (e.g., mesencephalitic reticular activating system, planum temporale), but both the N1 and P2 components are assumed to at least partially represent an exogenous response (see Crowley & Colrain, 2004 for review). On the other hand, N2 is believed to be an endogenous potential reflecting multiple neural processes associated with stimulus discrimination and classification (Näätänen, 1990). Specifically, N2 is associated with response inhibition in conflict tasks (Kopp, Rist, & Mattler, 1996), and reflects anterior cingulate cortex (ACC) activity (van Veen & Carter, 2002) related to action monitoring and evaluation during tasks requiring extensive executive control (Carter et al., 2000).

Magnié and colleagues (2000) found that the N1 and P2 components elicited during an auditory oddball task did not change after participants' body temperature and HR returned to baseline levels following maximal aerobic exercise. In addition, Nakamura and colleagues (1999) showed that

N1 during an auditory oddball task did not change 10 min after moderate exercise. These findings suggest that earlier exogenous components of the ERP may not be altered following acute aerobic exercise. In contrast, findings are mixed with respect to N2 changes after exercise. Themanson and Hillman (2006) investigated the effects of acute exercise on action monitoring using N2 during a modified flanker task. N2 occurs prior to response execution on correct trials and is thought to reflect response conflict (Kopp et al., 1996; Yeung, Cohen, & Botvinick, 2004). An increase in the allocation of attentional resources during stimulus updating following exercise (Hillman et al., 2003) would imply an increase in top-down attentional control (Themanson & Hillman, 2006). Accordingly, Themanson and Hillman (2006) predicted that less conflict monitoring would be needed following exercise and that a decrease in N2 amplitude would be observed. However, N2 did not change after participants' HR returned to baseline levels following moderately high aerobic exercise. In addition, Magnié and colleagues (2000) showed that N2 did not change after recovery of participants' body temperature following maximal exercise. Meanwhile, Duzova and colleagues (2005) indicated that N2 amplitude significantly decreased after recovery of participants' body temperature following maximal and short-duration (45 s) anaerobic exercise. From these findings, it is speculated that the effects of acute exercise on the N2 component may differ as a function of the exercise mode (i.e., aerobic or anaerobic).

Pontifex and Hillman (2007) observed smaller N1 and N2 amplitudes, larger P2 and P3 amplitudes, and longer N2 and P3 latencies with poorer task performance (i.e., lower accuracy) during exercise relative to rest. These data suggest that degradation of visual attention (i.e., smaller N1), increases in selective attention (i.e., larger P2), reduced ability to engage response inhibition (i.e., smaller N2), greater attentional resource allocation (i.e., P3 amplitude), and delayed processing speed (i.e., longer N2 and P3 latencies) may be observed during exercise. They further suggest that early deficits in stimulus acquisition may lead to inefficiency of cognitive processing despite attempts to increase top-down cognitive control, thus resulting in degradation of task performance (Pontifex & Hillman, 2007).

N400

Event-related potentials are also useful for the study of language comprehension because a negative component peaking around 400 ms after stimulus onset (N400) has been shown to vary systematically with the processing of semantic information (Kutas & Federmeier, 2000). Magnié and colleagues (2000) recorded the N400 component after participants' body temperature and HR returned to baseline levels following maximal cycling exercise. N400 amplitude, thought to be a general index of the ease or difficulty of retrieving stored conceptual knowledge associated with a word, is dependent on both the stored representation itself and the retrieval cues provided by the preceding context (van Petten & Luka, 2006). Magnié and colleagues (2000) indicated that N400 amplitude was significantly larger after acute exercise, suggesting that N400 changes may be caused by the general arousal effects of maximal aerobic exercise.

Contingent Negative Variation

Kamijo and colleagues (2004a) investigated the influence of exercise intensity on arousal level using the CNV. Contingent negative variation develops during the time interval between a warning stimulus and an imperative stimulus. It has been associated with psychophysiological events including expectancy (Walter et al., 1964), motivation (Irwin, Knott, McAdam, & Rebert, 1966), and attention and arousal (Tecce, 1972; Tecce, Savignano-Bowman, & Meinbresse, 1976). A number of studies have demonstrated that CNV consists of at least two components, an early CNV reflecting an orienting response (Loveless & Sanford, 1974; Weerts & Lang, 1973) and a late CNV reflecting motor preparation (Chwilla & Brunia, 1991; van Boxtel & Brunia, 1994; Van Boxtel, Geraats, Van den Berg-Lenssen, & Brunia, 1993). In particular, the relationship between early CNV in the frontal region and arousal level has been extensively reported (Higuchi, Watanuki, & Yasukouchi, 1997; Higuchi, Watanuki, Yasukouchi, & Sato, 1997; Tecce, 1972; Tecce et al., 1976). It has been shown that the mechanism of early CNV generation involves the ascending reticular formation system, which is strongly related to arousal level (McCallum et al., 1973; Picton & Low, 1971).

Kamijo and colleagues (2004a) found that both early and late CNV amplitudes decrease after high-intensity exercise and increase after medium-intensity exercise in a similar manner to the P3 amplitude (figure 7.4). The findings for the early CNV suggest that arousal level is affected by changes in exercise intensity. Changes in the late CNV amplitude suggest that acute exercise influences motor preparation.

ERN and Pe

Themanson and Hillman (2006) investigated the effects of acute aerobic exercise on cognitive functioning during a flanker task by comparing behavioral and neuroelectric indices of action monitoring. The error-related negativity (ERN or error negativity: Ne) and error positivity (Pe), as well as behavioral measures, were obtained following 30 min of acute treadmill exercise or following 30 min of rest. The ERN is a component of the response-locked ERP elicited when participants commit errors in a RT task. It is thought to reflect neuroelectric indices of action monitoring through a cognitive learning mechanism used to correct incorrect responses

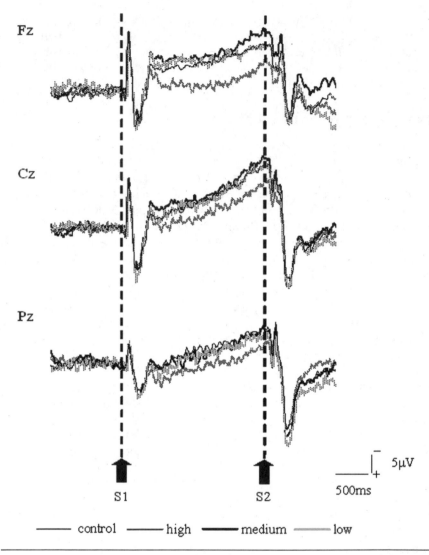

Figure 7.4 Grand averaged contingent negative variation waveforms from the Fz, Cz, and Pz electrode sites for all conditions (control condition and after low-, medium-, and high-intensity exercise).

Adapted from *Clinical Neurophysiology*, vol 115, K. Kamijo, Y. Nishihira, A. Hatta, T. Kaneda, T. Kida, T. Higashiura, and K. Kuriowa, "Changes in arousal level by differential exercise intensity," pgs. 2693-2698. Copyright 2004, with permission from Elsevier.

(Holroyd & Coles, 2002) or response conflict (Yeung et al., 2004). Pe is a late positive component occurring after the ERN response. The Pe has been described as an emotional reaction to the commission of an error (Falkenstein, Hoormann, Christ, & Hohnsbein, 2000; van Veen & Carter,

2002), as a postresponse evaluation of an error (Davies, Segalowitz, Dywan, & Pailing, 2001), and as the allocation of attentional resources following error commission (Mathewson, Dywan, & Segalowitz, 2005).

As with N2, Themanson and Hillman (2006) hypothesized that a reduction in response conflict associated with task execution (i.e., reduced ERN amplitude) would be observed following exercise because top-down attentional control would be increased. Further, they predicted that acute exercise may also influence Pe amplitude (Themanson & Hillman, 2006) because the Pe amplitude may reflect the allocation of attention toward an error in a manner similar to that during stimulus processing of correct trials (Mathewson et al., 2005). However, they found that all measures of cognitive function (e.g., ERN, Pe, RT, and accuracy) remained unchanged following acute exercise.

In summary, the effects of acute exercise on ERPs vary as a function of the stage of information processing in the central nervous system. Following acute exercise, earlier ERP components (exogenous potentials) seem to be less affected. Endogenous components such as N400 and CNV appear to be more influenced by acute exercise. However, ERN and Pe reflect action monitoring that does not appear to change following exercise.

Concluding Comments: Speculations About the Effects of Acute Exercise on ERP Indices of Cognitive Processing in Older Adults

Virtually all studies investigating the relationship between acute exercise and ERPs have focused on young adults, and data are not available regarding the effect of advancing age on these relationships. In this section, we speculate about the effects of advancing age on the relationship between acute exercise and ERP indices of cognitive processing.

Duzova and colleagues (2005) and Magnié and colleagues (2000) found that aerobic fitness levels do not influence ERP indices of cognitive function associated with acute aerobic exercise. These data suggest that age-related declines in fitness need not necessarily result in altered ERP responses. Furthermore, these researchers showed that P3 amplitude and latency at rest (i.e., preexercise) did not differ as a function of physical fitness levels. Several studies have addressed the relationship between long-term physical activity (i.e., chronic exercise) and P3 both in older and in younger adults. Data from these studies suggest that long-term physical activity is related to increased P3 amplitude and decreased P3 latency in older adults (Hatta et al., 2005; Hillman et al., 2004; Hillman, Kramer, Belopolsky, & Smith, 2006; Hillman, Weiss, Hagberg, & Hatfield, 2002), but these relationships are less clear in younger individuals (Hillman et al., 2006); this suggests that the effects of chronic exercise on ERPs in younger adults might be relatively smaller than in older adults. Studies are needed to examine whether acute exercise also influences ERP responses in older adults to a greater degree than in younger adults.

A number of studies have examined the effects of age and acute exercise on behavioral indices of performance in response to cognitive processing tasks. Using the Mini-Mental State Examination and a logical memory test, Molloy and coworkers (1988) found that cognitive performance in older adults (mean = 66 years) improved after 45 min of moderate-intensity exercise. In addition, Stones and Dawe (1993) reported that semantically cued memory in older adults (mean = 85 years) was significantly improved after 15 min of relatively low-intensity exercise. Emery and colleagues (2001) investigated the effects of acute exercise (about 35 min: 20 min maximal cycling exercise + 15 min cooling down) on cognitive function in both healthy older adults (mean = 69 years) and older patients with chronic obstructive pulmonary disease (COPD; mean = 68 years). They found that acute exercise was associated with improved performance on a verbal fluency test, a measure of verbal processing, only in the COPD patients, suggesting that acute exercise may benefit cognitive performance among COPD patients (Emery et al., 2001).

In conclusion, evidence from behavioral studies suggests that cognitive function in older adults may be facilitated after acute exercise. However, there is a need to extend this research to studies that measure the various components of ERP discussed in this chapter.

CHAPTER 8

Effects of Hormone Replacement Therapy on the Brains of Postmenopausal Women

A Review of Human Neuroimaging Studies

Kirk I. Erickson, PhD
Department of Psychology, University of Illinois at Urbana-Champaign

Donna L. Korol
Department of Psychology, University of Illinois at Urbana-Champaign

In this review we outline and synthesize the neuroimaging research that examines the effects of hormone therapy in postmenopausal women. On the basis of findings from preclinical and clinical studies, we predicted that a review of this literature would reveal that (a) hormone replacement has substantial effects on brain morphology, brain function, and cerebral blood flow and metabolism, as well as neurochemical, receptor, and metabolite concentrations; (b) effects of hormone therapy need to be interpreted within a multifactorial framework that includes age of the participants, age of menopause, duration of therapy, and time between onset of menopause and treatment initiation; and (c) effects of hormone therapy are relatively regionally specific. We argue that the extant neuroimaging literature on this topic supports all three of our predictions. That is, hormone therapy affects the brains of postmenopausal women but does so in a complex and multifactorial fashion, targeting some brain areas and neural mechanisms but not others. Future work and interpretations should take into account the burgeoning field of neuroimaging to assess the impact of hormone therapy on cognitive and brain health in women.

In humans, aging is often characterized by declining cognitive function, regional cortical volume loss, and altered functioning of the subsisting tissue. However, decay and deterioration in the brain and cognition are not ubiquitous facets of aging. While some older adults display significant declines on measures of executive functioning, such as working memory, task coordination, and attentional control, others exhibit spared functioning well into late adulthood. The source of this variability among older adults remains a question of high interest to the study of neurobiology of aging. Do specific lifestyle or genetic factors promote decline while others act to protect neural and cognitive function? Nutritional supplementation (Calvaresi & Bryan, 2001; Fukui et al., 2002), aerobic exercise (Colcombe et al., 2004), cognitive and intellectual engagement (Erickson et al., 2007b), and participation in social activities (Schooler & Mulatu, 2001; Wilson et al., 2002) have received consistent support as being neuroprotective. The influence of factors such as endogenous or supplementary hormone levels has remained a greater source of debate. In this review, we focus on the impact that hormone replacement therapy (HRT) has on the brains of postmenopausal women.

Studies of HRT and cognitive function in postmenopausal women have produced disparate and controversial findings. Findings from cross-sectional studies have promoted the idea that hormone treatment enhances verbal memory performance and decreases risk for developing dementia in postmenopausal women (Maki et al., 2001; Miller et al., 2001; Sherwin, 2003). Meta-analyses and reviews have also reported a general trend for an improvement in verbal memory as well as other cognitive processes in postmenopausal women undergoing HRT (Hogorvorst et al., 2000; Sherwin, 2003; Zec & Trivedi, 2002). In addition, a few relatively small randomized trials showed a decreased risk for dementia and cognitive decline associated with the use of HRT (Duka et al., 2000; Sherwin, 2003). Therefore, until recently, HRT was commonly depicted as a protective treatment against cognitive decline and dementia. Results from large randomized clinical trials, most notably the Women's Health Initiative (WHI), have challenged this conclusion with reports that the use of HRT increased the risk for development of dementia and impaired memory performance (Rapp et al., 2003; Resnick et al., 2006a, 2006b; Shumaker et al., 2003, 2004). These disparate research findings, suggesting on the one hand that HRT may be neuroprotective or beneficial for memory and cognition and on the other hand that it may increase the risk for dementia and cognitive decline, sparked a controversy leading to speculations about reasons for the discrepancy.

Several possibilities have been proposed to explain the contradictory findings: (1) the timing of treatment initiation, (2) variability in study design, (3) variability in the cognitive tasks employed, and (4) interactions between hormone treatment and other lifestyle factors (e.g., fitness). We briefly discuss each of these points next.

First, according to some, there exists a critical period or window of opportunity soon after menopause for HRT to exert positive effects on cognitive and neural systems (see Henderson, 2006; Maki, 2006; Sherwin, 2006). In support of this, a recent study from the WHI indicated that the risk for cardiovascular disease increases with an increase in years between menopause and the initiation of hormone treatment (Rossouw et al.,

2007), suggesting that HRT use at or around the time of menopause may produce beneficial effects on physiological function. Cross-sectional studies often assess women who began hormone treatment soon after menopause, whereas randomized clinical trials infrequently match treatment and control groups on hormone exposure time or treatment initiation. This could be a significant factor in explaining the contradictory findings between cross-sectional and randomized designs. Second, biases and confounds in study design (e.g., observational, randomized trials) could artificially inflate or negate effects of HRT. For example, some women choose to take HRT to counteract osteoporosis, while others take HRT to reduce menopausal symptoms such as hot flushes. For still other women, menopausal symptoms are not severe enough to warrant the use of hormone therapy. These group differences in health status and motivation for HRT use could confound group differences in cross-sectional and nonrandomized comparisons. Many studies, but not all, statistically control for or match for potentially confounding variables.

Third, cognitive outcome measures and assessments used to evaluate effects of HRT vary in their capabilities to measure specific cognitive operations (Henderson, 2006). It is likely that hormone therapy does not influence all brain regions and cognitive processes equally (Sherwin, 2006), so some tasks may be more sensitive to detecting effects of HRT than are others. Investigations in randomized trials are often limited to global measures of cognition, and may overlook effects that are specific to certain cognitive operations. Therefore, it is imperative for studies to avoid generalizing beyond the limitations of their cognitive measures to all of cognition or to facets of cognition not measured by the tests employed. Fourth, the contradictory findings in the HRT literature could be related to variation in demographic factors or to interactions among other lifestyle factors that moderate the effects of HRT on the brain and cognition (Erickson et al., 2007a). For example, age and fitness levels have both been shown to moderate the effect of hormone therapy on the brain. Cross-sectional studies and randomized trials infrequently take such factors into account when assessing the effects of hormone therapy.

In sum, there are a variety of potential explanations for the contradictory findings between nonrandomized and randomized human trials. Neuroimaging techniques have become valuable tools to investigate the influence of HRT on the human brain that both complement and add to cognitive testing methods. It is likely that the use of imaging techniques to examine the effects of hormone therapy on the brains of postmenopausal women will provide additional insight into the HRT controversy. More than 30 neuroimaging studies published in peer-reviewed journals have examined the influence of HRT on brain structure and function in postmenopausal women. In this review, we summarize and synthesize the neuroimaging studies addressing the effects of HRT on the brains of postmenopausal women with the hope that this literature will shed light on the presently controversial arena of HRT use and cognitive and brain health.

In addition to outlining the neuroimaging studies, we propose that synthesizing the neuroimaging research on HRT will support three main hypotheses: (1) There are striking differences in brain structure, brain function, cerebral blood flow, cerebral glucose metabolism, and receptor and metabolite concentrations between women receiving HRT and women not receiving HRT; and (2) hormone therapy covaries with age at menopause, age at which treatment is initiated, duration of therapy, and fitness levels. Therefore, any effects of HRT on the brain need to be interpreted within a multifactorial model, and (3) the effects of HRT are not global but rather are specific to particular regions of the brain. This level of specificity suggests that global cognitive measures will be unlikely to reveal any effects of hormone treatment.

We begin the review by discussing results from studies examining the relationship between hormone treatment and structural and volumetric measures of the brain. We then discuss the results from studies examining the effects of HRT on functional neuroimaging measures, cerebral blood flow, glucose metabolism, receptor concentrations, and metabolite concentrations.

Cortical Structure and Volume

Aging is frequently characterized by cortical and subcortical deterioration in prefrontal, temporal, and parietal cortices (Raz & Rodrigue, 2006). Although the cellular and biochemical factors that account for the volumetric declines have not been entirely delineated, many of the volumetric changes are correlated with functional and cognitive decline, suggesting that such morphological changes can have a significant impact on behavioral performance. Nonhuman animal research shows that estradiol administration influences a variety of morphological properties of the brain including dendritic spine density (Gould et al., 1990), capillary development (for review see Krause et al., 2006), and cell proliferation and survival (Tanapat et al., 1999). Using high-resolution magnetic resonance imaging (MRI) techniques, the morphology of the human brain can be assessed as a function of HRT use. As will be discussed in this section, there is a large degree of variability and discordance among the pattern of results on the topic of HRT effects on human brain morphology. However, we believe that some of the variability might be explained by the regional specificity of the analyses—that is, the degree to which the morphological analyses assess particular cortical loci. From this perspective, we believe that measurements of global cortical atrophy or volume may be unable to detect regionally specific effects of HRT.

Studies Reporting Differences in Cortical Structure as a Function of HRT

Hormone therapy has been found to be associated with either greater cortical volume or less decline in cortical volume with advancing age. Furthermore, there is evidence that HRT affects the brain in a site-specific manner, with the most dramatic effects on cortical areas that are most vulnerable to age-related deterioration such as the prefrontal cortices. For example, in a longitudinal, nonrandomized design, 12 women taking HRT and 12 women not taking HRT were studied over a five-year period (Raz et al., 2004b). The authors manually traced six brain regions including the hippocampus, lateral prefrontal cortex, prefrontal white matter, primary visual cortex, fusiform cortex, and entorhinal cortex. The volume of each region did not differ between treatment groups at baseline, but those women receiving HRT showed less neocortical brain shrinkage over a five-year interval. This effect was most robust in areas shown to be most vulnerable to aging, including the prefrontal cortical areas, and was strongest in women who remained on HRT for at least five years.

Other studies have also reported that the effects of HRT in postmenopausal women are largest in the gray matter of the prefrontal cortical regions. For example, studies using voxel-based morphometry (VBM), a technique that examines tissue density or volume on a point-by-point basis throughout the brain, show that the effects of HRT are most evident in the prefrontal cortex (Erickson et al., 2005; Boccardi et al., 2006). In fact, in concordance with the manual tracing results already discussed (Raz et al., 2004b), Erickson and colleagues (2005) reported an important age × HRT interaction in the prefrontal and parietal cortices, indicating that the use of HRT reliably offset the volumetric loss associated with advancing age. These findings (Raz et al., 2004b; Erickson et al., 2005) highlight the importance of examining age and its impact on HRT effects and suggest that the effects of HRT on the brain might be either specific or most robust in the prefrontal cortex, a region highly susceptible to age-related shrinkage.

Hormone replacement therapy also seems to affect white matter volume and white matter lesions. In one study of a cross-sectional sample of 70 women currently using HRT and 140 women not using it, HRT use was associated with fewer white matter lesions in users compared to nonusers (Schmidt et al., 1996). This effect was inversely related to the duration of HRT use, such that fewer white matter lesions were associated with longer exposures to HRT, where mean exposure duration was 4.4 years. In a longitudinal study following six postmenopausal women for two to six years (Cook et al., 2002) the groups did not differ on any measure at baseline, but periventricular hyperintensities and ventricular cerebral spinal fluid volume showed a lower mean increase in women receiving HRT than in those women not receiving HRT. Thus, in this small sample, HRT effectively thwarted the development of more white matter lesions with advancing age. Regional analyses have also shown that HRT is related to sparing of white matter volume in the tracts surrounding the hippocampus (Erickson et al., 2005; Ha et al., 2006) and prefrontal regions (Raz et al., 2004b). Although studies examining white matter have often used different measures, analyses, and designs, they suggest that HRT may protect against age-related increases in the number of white matter lesions and decreases in white matter volume in postmenopausal women.

Subcortical structures such as the hippocampus have also been examined in relation to HRT use. Although some studies have failed to find differences in hippocampal volume between women taking and not taking HRT (Raz et al., 2004b; Sullivan et al., 2005; Low et al., 2006), a few other studies have indicated that postmenopausal women receiving HRT had larger hippocampi than did postmenopausal women not receiving HRT (Eberling et al., 2003; Hu et al., 2006; Lord et al., 2006). Using manual tracing methods, a significant positive correlation between hippocampal volume and treatment duration was found, such that longer durations were associated with larger hippocampi (Lord et al., 2006). Two VBM studies have also shown that women receiving HRT exhibited greater hippocampal volume than did women not receiving HRT (Erickson et al., 2005; Boccardi et al., 2006), with larger hippocampi corresponding to longer durations of hormone therapy (Erickson et al., 2005). These varied results on effects of HRT on the hippocampal region, with some studies showing positive correlations (Eberling et al., 2003; Erickson et al., 2005; Hu et al., 2006; Lord et al., 2006) and others reporting no correlations with HRT treatment (Raz et al., 2004a, 2004b; Eberling et al., 2004; Sullivan et al., 2005), suggest that various factors may contribute to the sensitivity of the hippocampus to HRT. However, it should be noted that the majority of these conflicting studies were cross-sectional and that the only longitudinal study was not a randomized trial (Raz et al., 2004b). Therefore, many factors could contribute to the variability among these studies, including variation in age at menopause, age at treatment initiation, fitness, and the duration of hormone treatment.

Based on several reports in humans and nonhuman animal models, the timing of hormone treatment may be a critical factor in determining its efficacy for promoting healthy cognition and brain function (Erickson et al., 2005; Gibbs & Gabor, 2003; Marriott et al., 2002). Some studies have shown that longer durations are related to greater cortical volume (Erickson et al., 2005; Lord et al., 2006; Raz et al., 2004b) or fewer white matter lesions (Schmidt et al., 1996), while others have reported either no effect of duration of treatment (Low et al., 2006) or a negative correlation between hormone treatment duration and cortical volume (Greenberg et al., 2006). A closer examination of these studies reveals that reports of positive correlations between cortical volume and HRT have average treatment durations shorter than 10 years (Schmidt et al., 1996), whereas reports of negative correlations have average treatment durations longer than 10 years (Greenberg et al., 2006). In a recent VBM study, hormone exposures shorter than 10 years were associated with greater cortical volume in prefrontal, subgenual, and parahippocampal regions than hormone exposures longer than 10 years or in women who had never taken HRT (see figure 8.1; Erickson et al., 2007a). Furthermore, those women with hormone treatments extending beyond 10 years exhibited greater cortical decay than did women who had never taken HRT. Thus, shorter durations (within 10 years) spared brain volume, while longer durations (greater than 10 years) deteriorated brain volume. Importantly, these results were statistically adjusted for age, age at menopause, socioeconomic status, and other potentially important confounding variables, thereby isolating the effects of duration of treatment per se.

Strengthening the possibility that HRT influences cognition, HRT duration was also correlated with the number of perseverative errors on the Wisconsin Card Sort Test (WCST), a frequently used measure of executive function (see figure 8.2; Erickson et al., 2007a). Similar to what was seen with the cortical volume measures described earlier, women who were taking HRT for longer than 10 years had more perseverative errors on the WCST, while women with shorter durations had fewer perseverative errors. In sum, duration of treatment was related to cortical volume and WCST performance, and there was a reliable correlation between WCST performance and cortical volume. These effects clearly depict an important relationship between duration of hormone treatment, cortical volume, and executive functioning and indicate that longer durations of treatment are quantitatively and qualitatively different from shorter durations of treatment. This could potentially explain the variable results across studies, pointing to hormone duration as one critical factor.

A second important finding from Erickson and colleagues (2007a) was that the duration of hormone treatment statistically interacted with another lifestyle factor known to influence cortical volume and function—aerobic exercise (see figures 8.1 and 8.2). Exercise has now been shown repeatedly to enhance cortical volume measures and learning and memory operations (Kramer & Erickson, in press). In older adults, the effects of aerobic exercise tend to be largest on executive functioning measures and prefrontal cortex volume. Importantly, aerobic exercise increases some of the same molecular markers as estradiol, such as brain-derived neurotrophic factor (BDNF), a molecule produced and secreted by neurons that is considered critical in learning, memory, and neurogenesis (Lu et al., 2005). In fact, two studies using rodents showed reliable interactions between exercise and estradiol administration on BDNF levels in the hippocampus of ovariectomized female rats, with rats receiving both treatments having higher BDNF levels than rats receiving either treatment alone (Berchtold et al.,

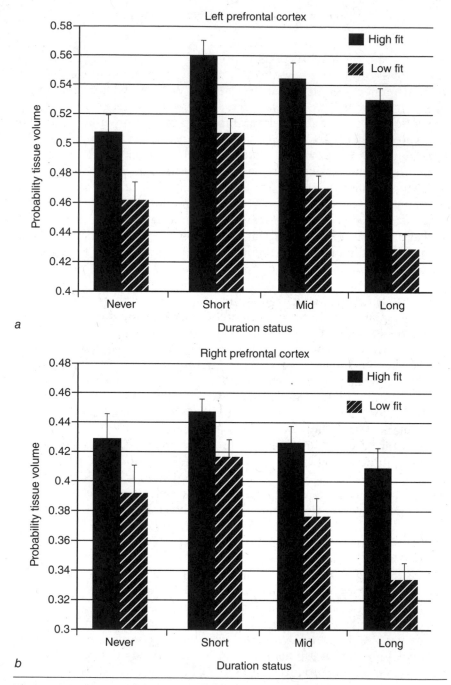

Figure 8.1 Mean volume measures in *(a)* left prefrontal cortex, *(b)* right prefrontal cortex, *(c)* left parahippocampal gyrus, and *(d)* subgenual cortex for never users, short-term users (<10 years), midterm users (10-15 years), and long-term users (>15 years) of hormone therapy. The solid bars represent aerobically high-fit participants and striped bars represent aerobically low-fit participants. *(continued)*

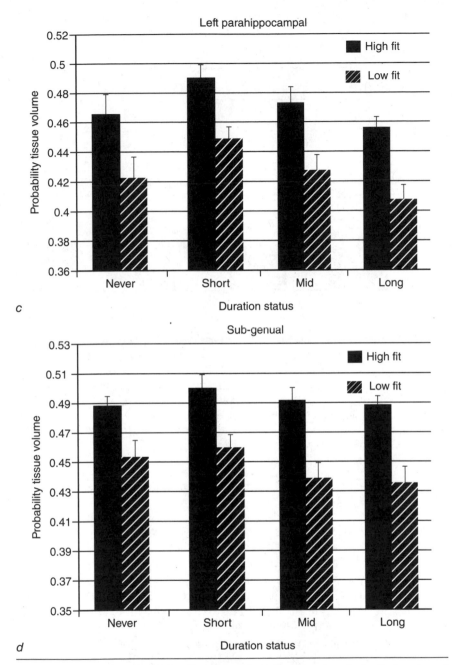

Left parahippocampal

c

Sub-genual

d

Figure 8.1 *(continued)* Main effects were found in all regions for both duration of treatment and fitness level. Interactions between fitness and duration of hormone treatment were found for the left and right prefrontal cortices. Both the left and right prefrontal regions were correlated with the number of perseverative errors on the Wisconsin Card Sort Test.

Adapted from *Neurobiology of Aging,* vol 28(2), K.I. Erickson, S.J. Colcombe, S. Elavsky, E. McAuley, E. Korol, P.E. Scalf, and A.F. Kramer, "Interactive effects of fitness and hormone treatment on brain health in postmenopausal women," pgs 179-185. Copyright 2007, with permission from Elsevier.

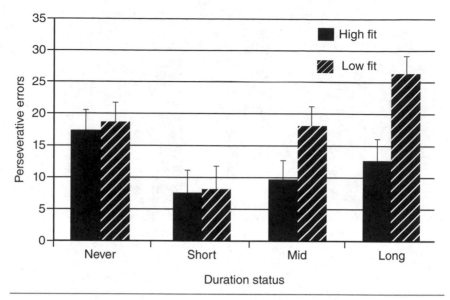

Figure 8.2 Adjusted means and standard errors for the number of perseverative errors on the Wisconsin Card Sort Test for never users, short-term users (<10 years), midterm users (10-15 years), and long-term users (>15 years) of hormone therapy. The solid bars represent participants with high aerobic fitness and the striped bars participants with low aerobic fitness. Long durations showed a significant increase in the number of perseverative errors, but this was reversed if long durations were accompanied by high aerobic fitness levels.

Adapted from *Neurobiology of Aging*, vol 28(2), K.I. Erickson, S.J. Colcombe, S. Elavsky, E. McAuley, E. Korol, P.E. Scalf, and A.F. Kramer, "Interactive effects of fitness and hormone treatment on brain health in postmenopausal women," pgs 179-185. Copyright 2007, with permission from Elsevier.

2001; Erickson et al., 2006). Moreover, the same exercise and estradiol regimens used to demonstrate changes in BDNF levels (Erickson et al., 2006) interact to improve rates of learning in a dual-solution maze task that can be solved with different cognitive strategies (Korol & Pruis, 2004). A meta-analysis of exercise interventions also revealed that the sex of the participant was a significant moderator of the effects of exercise on cognition (Colcombe & Kramer, 2003), again supporting the idea that aerobic exercise, or fitness levels, may interact with hormone status. As previously mentioned, aerobic exercise reliably offset the negative consequences of long durations of hormone treatment in postmenopausal women (Erickson et al., 2007a). Furthermore, exercise augmented the effects of short durations of hormone treatment. This effect was apparent not only in the VBM measures, but also in the number of perseverative errors on the WCST test. This interaction between multiple lifestyle factors is important as it highlights the interrelated nature of lifestyle factor influences on the brain that might account for significant variability within the hormone and exercise literatures. However, to date, no other known neuroimaging studies have investigated the relationship between hormone treatment and fitness levels.

In sum, the studies showing that HRT protects against age-related changes in cortical morphology largely utilize techniques such as VBM and manual tracing that allow regional analyses, and demonstrate the most dramatic effects in regions that exhibit the greatest degree of age-related cortical decline. Although there are a number of caveats about these techniques and their validity, convergence from multiple methods, labs, and populations strongly suggests that HRT has a significant impact on brain volume and white matter infarct severity.

Studies Failing to Find Differences in Cortical Structure as a Function of HRT

Most of the studies that fail to find differences in cortical volume as a function of HRT use measured global brain or lobar volume, which may not have spatial resolution sufficient for detecting regionally specific effects of HRT. For example, with use of a semiautomatic segmentation algorithm to separate tissue into gray and white matter, no differences in lobar gray or white matter volume between age-matched HRT users and nonusers were found (Resnick et al., 1998). Employing a similar technique for volumetric assessment, Sullivan and colleagues (2005) also reported no differences between HRT users and nonusers in the volume of the temporal lobe. It is important that both of these studies used a semiautomated technique and thus were not as susceptible to the confounds and reliability problems to which some other techniques are prone. However, it should be noted that both of these studies were cross-sectional, and the authors did not report controlling for potentially confounding lifestyle factors.

Those studies that involved regional analyses using manual tracing techniques often restricted assessments to the hippocampus and amygdala because of their involvement in dementia and aging (Low et al., 2006). It is possible that in humans the hippocampus is less susceptible to modulation by estradiol than are other areas such as the prefrontal cortical regions. For example, manually traced volumes of the hippocampus and amygdala did not differ between 213 HRT users and nonusers 60 to 64 years of age (Low et al., 2006). For measures of total brain volume, a measure of ventricle-to-brain ratio, and white matter hyperintensities, no differences between women receiving HRT and those not receiving HRT were found (Low et al., 2006). There were also no differences between current and past users of HRT or effects related to treatment duration (mean of 11.7 years for current HRT users and 5.0 years for previous HRT users). However, it is notable that these women were all within a very restricted age range, which could

143

have contributed to a lack of variability associated with age-related cortical decline and effects associated with HRT. However, other studies have also failed to find effects of HRT on manually traced hippocampal volume (Eberling et al., 2004; Raz et al., 2004a). Unlike other researchers using manual tracing, Low and colleagues (2006) did not manually trace cortical regions that are considered most susceptible to age-related deterioration (e.g., prefrontal cortex), which may have reduced the probability of finding effects of HRT on brain volume measures.

Not all studies involving assessment of specific regions show volume differences due to HRT use. In one cross-sectional study, the authors manually traced 13 cortical and subcortical regions and found no volumetric differences between women receiving HRT and women not receiving HRT (Raz et al., 2004a). This study, however, like the others already discussed, failed to adjust statistically for potentially confounding variables such as age at menopause or the duration of HRT use. Without statistical adjustment of potentially confounding variables, effects may be masked or may be driven by a correlated confounding factor.

Qualitative assessments of cortical atrophy have also been conducted; these studies show either no effect of HRT or greater subcortical atrophy with HRT use. For example, Luoto and colleagues (2000) qualitatively examined global brain atrophy, white matter hyperintensities, and infarcts in 2133 individuals characterized as either current, past, or never users of HRT. The authors reported that current users of HRT had greater central atrophy, represented by a higher ventricle-brain ratio, than either HRT-naïve women or past users of HRT. Unfortunately, the reliability and validity of qualitative assessments like that used by Luoto and colleagues (2000) are unknown. Greenberg and colleagues (2006) also found less cortical volume in women taking hormone therapy, but this study selected only women who had been taking HRT for over 10 years, with a mean duration of 23 years. As discussed previously, HRT durations longer than 10 years tend to be associated with greater cortical shrinkage.

Therefore, the majority of the data summarized in this section support the claim that the effects of HRT on cortical volume can be detected only through examination of particular areas of the brain (however, see Raz et al., 2004a for an exception).

Synthesis of Morphological and Volumetric Studies

In summary, 11 studies have indicated that HRT users have reduced infarct severity or greater cortical volume compared to their HRT-naïve counterparts; 5 studies have shown that HRT fails to affect brain volume measures; and 2 studies have demonstrated greater cortical atrophy in HRT users.

We proposed that measures with regional specificity would be more likely to show effects of HRT than would measures that assess only global cortical volume. Our review of the literature clearly supports this hypothesis, since four of the five studies failing to find differences were global, with the greatest degree of regional specificity limited to lobar measurements. In contrast, the majority of studies indicating that HRT spares brain volume or reduces infarct severity assessed cortical volume in a regionally specific fashion—and tended to focus on prefrontal cortical regions. Evidence for HRT effects on hippocampal volume in humans has not beeen as consistent, although in nonhumans, estradiol has been found to increase dendritic spine density and to boost other markers of neural plasticity in the hippocampus. Five studies showed that HRT was related to increased hippocampal volume (Boccardi et al., 2006; Eberling et al., 2003; Erickson et al., 2005; Hu et al., 2006; Lord et al., 2006) while an equal number of studies indicated that hippocampal volume did not differ as a function of HRT (Eberling et al., 2004; Low et al., 2006; Raz et al., 2004a, 2004b; Sullivan et al., 2005). The reasons for these contradictory findings on the hippocampus are unknown but could involve a variety of factors, including volumetric covariation with unassessed variables such as exercise or hormone duration (Erickson et al., 2007a) or population-related effects such as preclinical forms of dementia that are thought to influence the hippocampus more than other brain structures.

There is also a large degree of methodological inconsistency among the studies evaluating volumetric changes. Most studies are cross-sectional, and only a few statistically adjusted or matched for potentially confounding factors. Furthermore, although several studies have examined correlations with cognitive performance (e.g., Erickson et al., 2007a), very few consistently do so. Therefore, the relationship, or lack thereof, with cognitive and memory function is virtually unknown; and as previously discussed, correlations between neuroimaging measures and cognitive performance are critical for determining the behavioral importance of the neural effects of HRT.

Together the findings suggest that hormone treatment influences cortical morphology in a regionally specific manner, with the greatest effects in areas that are the most vulnerable to age-related deterioration such as the prefrontal cortex. Some of these effects are correlated with cognitive function and vary with the exposure time to the treatment.

Functional Neuroimaging

Positron emission tomography (PET) and functional MRI (fMRI) techniques have been used to examine functional characteristics of the human brain in a variety of contexts and populations. For example, older adults frequently exhibit impaired cortical function that is often correlated with cognitive performance deficits (e.g., Colcombe et al., 2005). People with

Alzheimer's dementia (AD) and mild cognitive impairment also experience abnormal patterns of activity during task performance, but these deficits can be partially improved through pharmaceutical treatments such as cholinesterase inhibitors (Goekoop et al., 2004). Other treatments such as six months of aerobic exercise (Colcombe et al., 2004) or cognitive training regimens (Erickson et al., 2007b) can significantly ameliorate age-related functional deficits and improve behavioral performance. In postmenopausal women, hormone treatments and interventions have been shown to improve cognitive function and mood perhaps through enhanced or altered brain activity.

All of the work described in this section clearly shows that hormones alter the pattern of cortical activity during verbal, spatial, figural, and odd-ball tasks as well as erotic video presentation. For example, in a study of the effects of HRT on cortical function during performance of a verbal and figural delayed-recognition memory test, women receiving HRT compared to HRT-naïve women performed better on the verbal and figural recognition memory tasks and showed altered patterns of activity in a network of brain areas thought to subsume memory operations, including prefrontal, parahippocampal, and precuneus regions (Resnick et al., 1998). However, the HRT-related changes in the processing of these areas were not simple monotonic increases or decreases in activity. Instead, the results revealed a complex pattern of change; some areas increased in activity with hormone use and other areas decreased in activity with hormone use. One caveat regarding this study, however, was the cross-sectional design. To overcome the design limitation, the authors followed some of these same participants over a two-year interval and rescanned them during performance of the same tasks (Maki & Resnick, 2000). In contrast to findings from the cross-sectional study, the longitudinal assessment demonstrated that women receiving HRT consistently showed increased activity in temporal, hippocampal, and parahippocampal regions over time (Maki & Resnick, 2000). Although no reliable improvements in behavior were reported, the increase in activity was interpreted as representing a more efficient use of the memory circuit during the task.

Recent findings obtained through use of a double-blind crossover design also suggest that the effects of HRT are not unidirectional (Shaywitz et al., 1999). The authors of this small double-blind randomized 21-day clinical trial studied 46 participants between the ages of 33 and 61, using fMRI to examine cortical activity during a verbal and a nonverbal working memory task. Similar to the results from the cross-sectional PET study (Resnick et al., 1998), hormone treatment was related to increased activity during verbal memory and decreased activity during nonverbal memory in some regions. Thus, while no improvements in behavioral performance were seen, the overall pattern of results suggests that HRT may alter functional patterns of activity during task performance, perhaps modifying the strategy used. This idea has been proposed, tested, and supported in rodents (see Korol, 2004).

More recent investigations have also shown consistent increases in brain activity during verbal and spatial working memory tasks in women taking HRT compared to their HRT-naïve peers (Joffe et al., 2006; Smith et al., 2006). In a double-blind 12-week trial, women on HRT experienced a greater increase in prefrontal activity for a spatial memory task, as well as a greater increase in the parietal and frontal cortices for a verbal memory task, than women not taking HRT (Joffe et al., 2006). In another study, a double-blind placebo-controlled crossover design using four-week intervals in conjunction with fMRI was employed to assess the effects of hormone therapy on brain activity during a spatial working memory task (Smith et al., 2006). In a double-blind 12-week trial in fifty-two women, women on HRT experienced a greater increase in the prefrontal activity for a spatial memory task, as well as a greater increase in the parietal and frontal cortices for a verbal memory task, than women not taking HRT (Joff et al., 2006). Again these effects were not correlated with improved spatial memory performance.

Hormone replacement therapy may also influence the pattern of brain activity during tasks that involve either attentional control or physiological arousal. Hormone effects on brain activity of 16 older women (ages 73-84) during an oddball task requiring high attentional control suggest that HRT was associated with increased activity in some regions and decreased activity in other regions that are often implicated in perception and attention processes (Stevens et al., 2005). These effects were interpreted as representing a hormone-induced increase in neural efficiency during attention and vigilance tasks. Finally, neural correlates of hormone-induced changes in sexual arousal and cognitive and emotional function in postmenopausal women have been found (Archer et al., 2006). Specifically, only under combined estradiol and testosterone therapy were levels of limbic cortical activity similar to those of premenopausal women, yet estradiol therapy alone was related to increased levels of activity compared to no-hormone treatment.

Thus, hormones clearly alter cortical function as assessed by PET and fMRI. The direction and behavioral implications of these results are less clear. Many of the studies describe both increases and decreases in activity, and none have shown that these changes are correlated with improved cognitive or emotional function. Until correlations with behavioral performance can be derived, the impact of the altered pattern of brain activity remains speculative. One hypothesis is that group differences in brain activity represent different cognitive strategies undertaken while hormone therapy is being received (Korol, 2004). In addition, because of the expense of PET and fMRI, these studies typically have small sample sizes, thus precluding the capability to do correlation analyses. Furthermore, the wide range of ages used in these studies (from 33 to 84) could contribute to a large degree of variation regarding the efficacy of hormone treatment in moderating functional patterns of brain activity. It is possible that the effects of HRT on cognition and brain function are sensitive to age-related declines, with the greatest effects of HRT found in aged populations.

Despite some limitations, emerging from this literature is important support for the argument that hormones influence brain activity. Most of the designs are longitudinal, clinically randomized, or crossover and are thus less susceptible to many of the limitations of cross-sectional designs. In addition, all studies show increases in activity, and most show that this effect has a locus around the prefrontal cortex—an area also heavily implicated in cognitive function and age-related cognitive decline. Thus, functional neuroimaging results support claims that HRT influences brain function, perhaps in a regionally specific manner.

Resting Regional and Global Cerebral Blood Flow

Resting regional cerebral blood flow (CBF) decreases in healthy elderly persons (Bentourkia et al., 2000; Martin et al., 1991; Melamed et al., 1980) and even more so in patients with AD (Bonte et al., 1986; Eberling et al., 1992; Montaldi et al., 1990). In fact, the severity of dementia and cognitive deficits is negatively correlated with global resting CBF values (Bartenstein et al., 1997; Eberling et al., 1993), with resting CBF values thought to be a reliable diagnostic marker of early AD (Nobili et al., 2001; Prohovnik et al., 1988). In fact, in both cross-sectional and longitudinal studies (Hogh et al., 2001; Sakamoto et al., 2003; Tanaka et al., 1998), people with a genetic risk for developing AD who have not yet presented any symptoms also exhibit decreased resting CBF. Decreases in resting CBF are most evident in the temporal-parietal cortex and the frontal cortex, areas that are considered important components of a memory circuit affected by aging and pathology (Buckner et al., 2005). Furthermore, some treatments, such as acetylcholinesterase inhibitors, alleviate the CBF deficits in AD patients (Nobili et al., 2002; Staff et al., 2000), suggesting that CBF can be used not only as a marker of decline, but also as a measure of treatment efficacy.

Early evidence that hormone therapy decreases the risk for developing AD prompted researchers to examine whether HRT would act through changes in CBF in postmenopausal women to protect against developing AD. The first of these studies examined resting CBF by using an ^{133}Xe inhalation technique in 158 postmenopausal women, of whom 51 had a history of cerebrovascular disease (Funk et al., 1991). In an observational study over an 18-month period, the authors reported that only in women with a history of cerebrovascular disease was HRT related to an increase in resting CBF; those women not receiving treatment showed no change. The authors statistically adjusted for time since menopause but did not control for or report the influence of other potentially confounding factors such as socioeconomic status, form and dose of treatment, or age at menopause.

Subsequent studies employed single-photon emission computed tomography (SPECT) to examine resting CBF. In a nonrandomized trial, 9 of 14 women were assigned to hormone treatment for a two- or three-week period (Ohkura et al., 1995). The treatment and control groups showed similar resting CBF levels at baseline, but the group receiving hormone therapy showed significant increases in cerebral and cerebellar blood flow. Similar hormone-induced increases in resting CBF were reported in two other SPECT studies that assigned women to either six weeks of estrogen treatment (Greene, 2000) or one year of estrogen treatment (Slopien et al., 2003). These studies all indicated that hormone treatment, even in relatively acute doses of two or three weeks, produced enhanced resting global CBF values. Despite the consistent results, one limitation of both ^{133}Xe inhalation and SPECT techniques is their poor spatial resolution. PET is another technique that provides a measure of resting CBF that has higher spatial resolution and thus provides increased regional specificity and allows for better localization of changes.

In one study employing a cross-sectional design, there were no differences in resting regional CBF between HRT users and nonusers (Resnick et al., 1998). However, in a two-year follow-up, HRT users exhibited an increase in resting regional CBF in the left and right temporal lobe while the group not receiving HRT showed no changes in CBF (Maki & Resnick, 2000). The differences in study design (longitudinal vs. cross-sectional) highlight the possible confounds associated with cross-sectional designs, such as baseline differences in CBF that obstruct the accurate assessment of effects of hormone treatment.

Together, the results from these studies—using a variety of imaging techniques to examine CBF—argue that HRT administration, at least in longitudinal assessments, increases CBF in postmenopausal women. Whether increased CBF is influencing the fMRI results discussed previously is currently not known, but the possibility remains. All of the studies we have described were limited to women without any known pathology. It has been argued that the cognitive and neural deterioration accompanying dementia differs fundamentally in the molecular processes and the trajectory of cortical decay from declines associated with nondemented older adults (Buckner et al., 2005). Because of AD-related decline in cognitive and neural function, HRT may have more dramatic effects on outcome measures in a dysfunctional population.

Despite the possibility that dysfunction may increase the likelihood of HRT effects, evidence is mixed regarding the impact of HRT on resting CBF in women who have been diagnosed with AD or probable AD. Ohkura and colleagues (1994) studied 15 AD patients using SPECT in a nonrandomized HRT intervention for four to six weeks. They found that AD patients taking HRT displayed a reliable increase in resting CBF. However, Wang and colleagues (2000), who studied 50 women diagnosed with AD in a randomized double-blind placebo trial for 12 weeks, failed to find any changes in resting CBF after hormone treatment.

There is a high degree of consistency among the results outlined in this section. All of the studies, except for one cross-sectional study (Resnick et al., 1998) and one study with AD patients (Wang et al., 2000), have shown increased resting regional or global CBF with hormone treatment. Therefore, the results from these studies suggest that HRT can have a significant impact on resting CBF. Given that resting CBF decreases with both healthy and pathological aging and is considered an important marker of cognitive and neural decline, a hormone-induced increase in resting CBF may mark improved brain function.

Importantly, these results and interpretations in the studies outlined here also withstand an amazing degree of methodological inconsistency. For example, the mean age in the samples ranges between 44 and 67 (and 72 in the AD patients), while time between menopause and treatment is rarely assessed or controlled. As already mentioned, the length of time between menopause and the onset of hormone treatment is now considered an important factor because with increasing time after menopause, the effects of HRT may dissipate or even become detrimental (Rossouw et al., 2007). Given the large amount of variability in the mean age of the samples, the fact that none of the studies reviewed addresses or statistically controls for time between menopause and treatment initiation is an important limiting factor. In addition, the duration of treatment in the longitudinal and intervention studies ranges from two weeks to two years, and the statistics focus on within-group comparisons, rarely considering time × group interactions. Furthermore, many of the intervention studies are nonrandomized or fail to use control groups, and matching or controlling for confounding factors such as age and years of education is rare. Finally, many of these reports omit correlations with cognitive or behavioral outcomes yet assume improved behavioral function, whether it be cognitive, emotional, or social, associated with increased resting CBF. Particularly in light of these limitations, the CBF results are amazingly consistent and argue for robust and reliable effects of hormone treatment on CBF.

Cerebral Glucose Metabolism

Given the neuroprotective evidence for estradiol, some studies have investigated whether HRT could also alter the pattern of glucose metabolism in healthy, nondemented postmenopausal women. Similar to research on resting CBF, studies that examine cerebral glucose metabolism by employing 2-deoxy-2-[^{18}F]fluoro-D-glucose (FDG)-PET have consistently shown lower regional metabolic rates in AD patients (e.g., Friedland et al., 1983).

In fact, middle-aged people with the apolipoprotein-ε4 allele exhibit a greater magnitude of metabolic decline over two years than do those without an ε4 allele (Small et al., 1995, 2000). Furthermore, the proportion of cognitive impairment in pathological populations is positively related to hypometabolism in certain brain regions including the precuneus, posterior cingulate, and retrosplenial cortex (Buckner et al., 2005). Some treatments, such as acetylcholinesterase inhibitors, produce increased metabolism in the cortical circuitry involved in memory (Mega et al., 2001; Nordberg et al., 1992; Potkin et al., 2001).

A relatively small set of studies using measures of glucose metabolism has consistently shown that HRT use is associated with higher metabolic rates compared to those in nontreated women. In one cross-sectional study, after age and years of education were controlled, women receiving HRT exhibited greater glucose metabolism in the dorsolateral prefrontal cortex, middle temporal gyrus, and inferior parietal lobule than did untreated women and women diagnosed with AD (Eberling et al., 2000). In another cross-sectional study, compared to HRT users, women receiving the selective estrogen receptor modulator tamoxifen, which has both estrogen receptor agonist and antagonist actions, as well as women not receiving any treatment, had glucose hypometabolism throughout the frontal and prefrontal cortices but not in the hippocampus (Eberling et al., 2004). Unfortunately, the duration of treatment was approximately 17 years for women in the HRT group and approximately two years in the tamoxifen group, a potentially significant confound. Semantic memory performance was also poorer for tamoxifen users than for the other groups, but this effect was not correlated with differences in metabolism. While the results from both of these studies suggest that HRT use is related to higher glucose metabolism, their cross-sectional character precludes any causal claims about HRT use. Similar to what is seen with other cross-sectional designs, potential confounding variables such as a healthy-user bias could have contributed to some of the effects. For example, women who choose to take HRT may be inherently healthier than women who choose not to take HRT. Concern for their health, as well as economic capabilities to obtain HRT, could also systematically differ between women who choose to take HRT those who choose not to.

Longitudinal studies also show effects of HRT on glucose metabolism, yet the regions most affected by hormone treatment in longitudinal studies are different from those affected in cross-sectional studies. In one study, conducted over a two-year interval, four postmenopausal women receiving HRT and six postmenopausal women not receiving HRT were statistically matched for parity, mean age at menopause, length of reproductive life, and body mass index (Rasgon et al., 2001). The authors reported that HRT users showed a significant increase in glucose metabolism in the lateral temporal lobe, while men and nonusers showed no alteration in metabolism over two years. In a follow-up two-year longitudinal study using a slightly larger sample, Rasgon and colleagues (2005) reported a reliable decrease in glucose metabolism in the posterior cingulate in nonusers, with no reliable decrease in glucose metabolism over the two-year period in HRT users. Although the results from these studies were interpreted similarly, they were qualitatively different. In the first study, HRT use was associated with an increase in metabolism, whereas in the second it was associated with a sparing of metabolism from decline rather than an increase per se. Therefore, the direction of the effect was quite different in the two studies; but because declines in glucose metabolism are associated with both AD and age-related cognitive decline, increases in and sparing of glucose metabolism with HRT use are both interpreted as reflective of a neuroprotective characteristic of hormone treatment. These two studies, however, indicated that the locus of HRT effects was in the posterior cingulate and medial temporal cortex—regions commonly implicated in metabolic deficits in AD patients but differing from the dorsolateral prefrontal areas implicated in cross-sectional studies (Eberling et al., 2000, 2004).

Studies examining the effects of HRT on glucose metabolism have consistently reported either increased or spared metabolism over a two-year interval in postmenopausal women taking HRT. However, despite this consistency, a number of critical limitations prohibit definitive conclusions about the effects of HRT on glucose metabolism. For example, each of the four studies had a small sample size, making generalizations to the population difficult. In addition, the neuroanatomical locus of the difference in metabolism between the groups varied, with cross-sectional studies showing the largest effects of HRT on prefrontal cortex metabolism and longitudinal studies showing the largest effects in the posterior cingulate cortex. However, despite these limitations, the results indicate that hormone therapy is associated with increased cerebral glucose metabolism.

Serotonin Receptor and Cholinergic Terminal Concentrations

Hormones may modulate emotional and cognitive function through neurotransmission modulation. In rodents, estradiol acts to modulate both the production of proteins and the release of neurochemicals from the synapse that could in turn influence cognition and behavior. Modulation of serotonin receptor ($5\text{-}HT_{2A}$) concentrations in the anterior cingulate and frontal cortex has been found following treatment with estradiol (Cyr et al., 1998; Sumner & Fink, 1997). Furthermore, estradiol is thought to enhance cognitive function at least partly through the regulation of cholinergic function, including acetylcholinesterase levels and acetylcholine release in the hippocampus, cortex, and basal forebrain of rats (Gibbs et al., 1997; Korol & Marriott, 2003; Luine et al., 1980). Therefore, due to the strong neuromodulatory role of estrogens on neurotransmitters and receptors, a number of studies have examined whether HRT use in women is associated with increased concentrations of 5-HT$_{2A}$ receptors and cholinergic terminals.

The 5-HT$_{2A}$ receptor is frequently studied in vivo in the human brain because it is one of the few receptors with a radioactive ligand that can be imaged using PET. In rodents, the [^{18}F]altanserin ligand has a high affinity and is very selective for 5-HT$_{2A}$ receptors (Lemaire et al., 1991); its imaging with PET is comparable to in vitro mapping of 5-HT$_{2A}$ receptors (Biver et al., 1997). In the human brain, the [^{18}F]altanserin ligand has a robust test–retest reliability (Smith et al., 1998) and is frequently used to study depression and schizophrenia (e.g., Mintun et al., 2004). Although 5-HT$_{2A}$ receptors are infrequently studied in age-related pathologies such as AD, there has been one report of reduced 5-HT$_{2A}$ receptor density in healthy elderly subjects (Meltzer et al., 1998).

Although only a few studies on this issue have been conducted, it is apparent that HRT is consistently associated with increased 5-HT$_{2A}$ concentrations and cholinergic synaptic terminal density in a few areas of cortex including the prefrontal and parietal cortices. For example, Moses and colleagues (2000) examined five postmenopausal women at multiple time points: baseline before treatment, after 8 to 14 weeks of estrogen replacement, and then again after 2 to 6 weeks of combined estrogen plus progesterone. The authors found widespread increases in receptor binding throughout the cerebral cortex, but only following the combination of estrogen and progesterone treatment. Moses-Kolko and colleagues (2003) extended this effect to a voxel-based measurement approach that can assess receptor concentrations on a fine-grained scale throughout the brain. They reported that unopposed estrogen treatment increased 5-HT$_{2A}$ receptor concentrations in the prefrontal cortex, parietal cortex, and temporal cortex above those of untreated women, and that the combination of estrogen and progesterone potentiated the estrogen-related increase in 5-HT$_{2A}$ receptor concentration. Kugaya and colleagues (2003) also showed increased 5-HT$_{2A}$ receptor binding in 10 postmenopausal women receiving unopposed estrogen treatment for 10 weeks. They reported that the change in receptor concentration in the inferior frontal cortex was correlated with plasma estradiol levels, yet behavioral improvements on cognitive measures were uncorrelated with the change in 5-HT$_{2A}$ receptor concentration.

The results from Moses and colleagues (2000) and Moses-Kolko and colleagues (2003) suggest that the effects of HRT may increase with longer exposures to estrogen. In support of this hypothesis, other markers of brain function have been related to the duration of hormone treatment. For example, Smith and colleagues (2001) examined the influence of long-term HRT use (mean ~15 years) on cholinergic synaptic concentrations in postmenopausal women using the radiotracer [^{123}I]iodo-benzovesamicol ([^{123}I]IBVM), which is a marker for vesicular acetylcholine transporter, an index of cholinergic synaptic terminal density (Kuhl et al., 1996). Although there were no main effects of HRT treatment, the length of hormone treatment was positively correlated with cholinergic binding indices in the frontal cortex, parietal cortex, temporal cortex, and anterior and posterior cingulate. Furthermore, the authors reported that the use of unopposed estrogen was associated with greater terminal concentrations in the posterior cingulate than the combination of estrogen and progesterone treatment.

The studies outlined did not indicate any correlation between receptor or terminal concentrations and emotional or cognitive performance, even though increases in receptor concentrations and cholinergic synaptic terminal density have been interpreted as benefiting cognitive and emotional functioning. It is possible that the increased concentrations need to be maintained for an extended period of time before any cognitive benefits are subsumed by the system, or simply that the cognitive tasks employed were not sensitive to the receptor concentration changes. The sample sizes in these studies are quite small, and correlations would need to be quite robust to detect any reliable relationship. Larger sample sizes would be more conducive to correlation analyses. However, regardless of these limitations, these studies suggest that HRT and the duration of treatment influence the effect of hormone use on receptor concentrations in a site-specific manner in the cortex, the largest effects occurring with longer durations in the prefrontal cortex.

Metabolite Concentrations

Because of its neuroprotective effects, HRT might be an effective modulator of metabolite concentrations in postmenopausal women. Brain injury and disease have been associated with increased metabolite levels as measured by magnetic resonance proton spectroscopy (Brooks et al., 2001). Higher metabolite concentrations have been found in older adults with and without dementia, and these effects sometimes correlate with impaired cognitive function (Chantal et al., 2004; Kantarci et al., 2002).

Only two studies to date, both cross-sectional in design, have examined the influence of HRT on metabolite levels; both report that HRT offset age-related changes in metabolite concentration. In one, Robertson and colleagues (2001) examined 24 young women, 21 postmenopausal long-term and current users of HRT, and 16 women who had never used HRT. The authors reported that the concentration of choline-containing compounds, considered to be markers of neuronal and glial membrane turnover, were significantly higher in the parietal lobe and hippocampus in HRT-naïve women compared to women receiving HRT and young women. These results suggest that HRT use is associated with reduced membrane turnover and thus less cellular deterioration. Although there were no correlations between choline levels and duration of hormone use or years since menopause, hippocampal choline levels were negatively correlated with long-term visual memory performance as measured by the Wechsler Memory Scale. This was one of the first studies to report a reliable correlation between neuroimaging measures and cognitive measures in postmenopausal women.

In addition, HRT use lowers an age-related increase in myo-inositol (MI) levels, thus resulting in a favorable modulation of brain aging. Ernst and colleagues (2002) failed to find an impact of HRT on choline-containing compounds but found lower concentrations of MI in the frontal white matter, basal ganglia, and hippocampus in women receiving estrogen compared to women who had never used HRT. Myo-inositol is considered a measure of glial content or activity (Brand et al., 1993), and higher MI levels are representative of poorer glial function, which can be observed in nonpathological aging (Chang et al., 1996). Ernst and colleagues (2002) also included a group of women receiving tamoxifen and reported that these women showed a reduction in MI levels similar to that in the participants receiving HRT. In addition, an inverse relationship was reported between basal ganglia MI levels and the duration of HRT use. The average duration of HRT for women in this study was 20 years, and the authors speculate that the effects of HRT on brain chemistry in the cortex may reach asymptote prior to 20 years of exposure.

Although both of these studies were cross-sectional and therefore prone to the same healthy-user bias and potential confounding limitations as any other cross-sectional study, they did have relatively large sample sizes (71 women in Robertson et al., 2001 and 76 women in Ernst et al., 2002). In addition, Robertson and colleagues (2001) found a significant correlation with metabolite levels and long-term visual memory performance, suggesting that these metabolite differences have a potentially important relationship to cognitive function. However, it is important to note that the metabolites affected by HRT were different between the two studies, revealing a source of inconsistency. In short, the evidence suggests that HRT may have some effect on metabolite concentrations; but which metabolites are most affected, as well as the relationship of these effects to cognition, have not been fully characterized.

Discussion

At the outset, we proposed that synthesizing the neuroimaging research on HRT would provide support for three separate hypotheses: (a) that there are striking differences in brain morphology, brain function, CBF, metabolism, and metabolite and receptor concentrations as a function of HRT; (b) that the influence of HRT on the brain must be interpreted within a multifactorial model that includes age at menopause, age at which treatment is begun, the duration of therapy, and the particular cognitive task being examined; and (c) that the effects of HRT are specific to particular regions of the brain, suggesting that global cognitive or neuroimaging measures would be unlikely to show any effects of hormone use.

Although some studies have reported small or insignificant effects of HRT on the brain, the majority have shown the opposite pattern: HRT has a considerable impact on brain volume, functional activity, blood flow, and receptor and metabolite concentrations. Despite a large degree of methodological inconsistency among studies, the results are strikingly similar in their overall pattern. In all circumstances the differences between HRT users and nonusers were interpreted as evidence that HRT benefits the postmenopausal brain, despite very few correlations between brain results and behavioral results. However, in many studies, HRT seemed to offset, or to slow, the negative consequences of aging on the brain, suggesting in fact that HRT is an important moderator of cortical aging. It is evident from this review that for definitive conclusions to be drawn, larger sample sizes in randomized designs and correlations with behavioral performance are needed.

Consistent with our second hypothesis, however, most studies indicate a complex relationship between HRT use and the brain. For example, it is clear that there exists a relationship between the duration of hormone therapy and certain brain measures and that this relationship is not necessarily linear (Erickson et al., 2007a). In fact, we have argued that hormone exposures greater than 10 years tend to show negative correlations with neuroimaging measures, whereas hormone exposures less than 10 years tend to show positive correlations. The duration of hormone therapy is clearly an important moderating factor for determining the positive and negative consequences of HRT on cognition and the brain. Although some authors have speculated about a critical window of opportunity for HRT to exert its effects (Sherwin, 2006), there have not been any neuroimaging studies that formally investigate this (however, see Lord et al., 2006). Some studies show interactions between HRT use and age and flatter slopes of cortical deterioration in longitudinal designs of HRT use (Erickson et al., 2005; Raz et al., 2004b). These effects provide some preliminary evidence for the existence of a window of opportunity in postmenopausal women (Erickson et al., 2005; Raz et al., 2004b). In addition, other lifestyle factors, such as exercise (Erickson et al., 2007a), influence the outcome and interpretations of HRT effects on the brain. In short, the effects of HRT should be interpreted cautiously and within a multifactorial framework. The question "Does HRT affect the brain?" should be rephrased to provide a transparent representation of this complexity—for example, to "What are the factors that limit or enhance the influence of HRT on the brain?"

The spatial resolution of the techniques employed also influences whether relationships between HRT and brain measures are detected. We predicted that the effects of HRT would be regionally specific and that techniques limited by poorer spatial resolution would fail to detect effects of HRT. Results from both functional and structural MRI studies, along with measures of receptor concentrations, strongly support this prediction. Specifically, prefrontal cortical areas display the greatest age-related deterioration, and it is these areas that show the most robust effects of HRT use. Importantly, this implies that cognitive measures that are global or that rely on cortical regions not affected by HRT, such as the prefrontal cortex, might fail to show an effect of hormone therapy. Erickson and colleagues (2007a) provide a clear example. In this study, the number of perseverative errors on the WCST varied with the duration of HRT use and also correlated with the volume of tissue in the prefrontal cortex. However, a commonly employed measure of global cognitive function, the Mini-Mental State Examination (MMSE), was unrelated to HRT use and was uncorrelated with brain volume measures.

There are also a number of limitations regarding the techniques and results discussed in this review. First, most of the studies were not randomized designs or even longitudinal designs; thus, it is unknown to what extent a healthy-user bias influenced the results. For example, women who choose to take HRT may differ systematically in their health status from women who choose not to. Furthermore, women who take HRT for longer durations usually do so for relief or treatment of health problems such as osteoporosis, whereas women who take HRT for shorter durations do so to relieve postmenopausal symptoms such as hot flushes. Therefore, health-related differences between groups could artificially amplify or negate results related to HRT use.

A second limitation of the studies discussed in this review is the lack of comparisons using multiple neuroimaging techniques within a particular population. For example, fMRI studies have yet to examine whether the differences reported are related to the volume or density of tissue within the activated or deactivated region. Since there is now evidence that HRT influences cortical volume, especially in the prefrontal regions, it is plausible that some of the variation in functional activity between HRT users and nonusers could be due to the volume of tissue within that region. This may influence interpretations of the effects of HRT on brain activation. For example, functional differences that are unrelated to the volume of tissue could be considered related to the efficiency of the processing within the region, whereas functional differences that are correlated with the volume of tissue in the region could be related to a general deterioration in cortical resources. Future neuroimaging research could investigate these possibilities.

In summary, the influence of HRT on the health of postmenopausal women will remain a controversial topic. However, this review suggests that some valuable results can be gleaned from the use of neuroimaging techniques. Although it may still be too early to discuss definitively the effects of HRT on the postmenopausal brain, it is likely that hormone therapy is a factor that could be grouped alongside other critical lifestyle factors that induce cortical plasticity such as aerobic exercise, nutritional supplementation, and intellectual engagement.

CHAPTER 9

Physical Activity Programming to Promote Cognitive Function

Are We Ready for Prescription?

Jennifer L. Etnier, PhD

Department of Exercise and Sport Science,
University of North Carolina at Greensboro

The empirical literature clearly demonstrates a positive relationship between physical activity and cognitive functioning, with meta-analytic reviews showing that the effect size ranges from small to moderate (Colcombe & Kramer, 2003; Etnier et al., 1997; Heyn, Abreu, & Ottenbacher, 2004; Sibley & Etnier, 2003). The evidence also suggests that these effects are larger for individuals who are at risk for cognitive decline either due to advancing age (Colcombe & Kramer, 2003; Etnier et al., 1997) or due to the experience of cognitive impairments (Heyn et al., 2004). Given the consistency with which physical activity has been shown to be associated with cognitive benefits, a natural and practical question is, "How much and what type of exercise should an individual perform in order to improve or protect cognitive abilities?" In other words, have dose–response relationships between physical activity and cognitive performance been established to a sufficient extent that we are ready to prescribe exercise as an intervention intended to facilitate improved cognitive performance?

In a recent consensus symposium, experts from around the world addressed the question of whether or not there is a dose–response relationship between physical activity and physical health, quality of life, and depression and anxiety (published in a supplement to *Medicine and Science in Sports and Exercise,* 2001). However, this same issue has not been addressed for the relationship between physical activity and cognitive performance. Thus, the purpose of this review is to provide an assessment of the existing evidence relative to the establishment of a dose–response relationship between physical activity and cognitive performance.

The aspects of physical activity that one must consider when examining dose–response relationships include mode, duration, intensity, frequency, and length of physical activity participation. Mode is often defined as the specific type of activity that a person is performing (e.g., swimming, bicycling, walking, upper-body strength training), and this information is needed to estimate the energy expenditure required for that activity. Duration is the amount of time spent in a single bout of physical activity. However, duration is complicated by the fact that effects on cognition may be influenced by whether the physical activity on a given day is completed in a single bout or is accumulated in multiple bouts over the course of the day. This is particularly relevant given the 1995 American College of Sports Medicine (ACSM) and the Centers for Disease Control (CDC) recommendation that, for health outcomes, adults should "accumulate" 30 or more min of exercise per day (minimum of 8 min bouts). In 1998, ACSM revised its recommendation with respect to duration (20-60 min), but maintained its position that the exercise could be performed continuously or intermittently (minimum of 10 min bouts). Intensity is reflective of the percent of maximal effort at which an individual is performing. Together, duration and intensity determine the total energy expenditure of an activity. Frequency refers to the number of days of physical activity per week and, when combined with intensity and duration, provides a measure of weekly volume of physical activity. The length of physical activity participation is typically expressed in weeks or months and may provide an indication of whether the effects of physical activity on cognition occur over a relatively short period of time or whether a longer commitment to activity is needed for benefits to accrue.

Evaluating the evidence regarding dose–response relationships is challenging in every research area, but particularly so in the area of physical activity and cognition. The strongest evidence for evaluating dose response would come from reviewing those randomized controlled trials (RCTs) that address the relationship using comparable techniques. However, in the area of physical activity and cognitive performance, a large body of RCTs does not exist and thus cannot be examined to determine whether or not there is a consistent pattern of results. In fact, in the area of physical activity and cognition, very few RCTs have been conducted at all; and to my knowledge, no large-scale RCT has examined dose–response issues relative to the relationship between physical activity and cognitive performance.

Given that the "gold standard" evidence is not available, other lines of evidence can be evaluated to determine whether or not we have sufficient knowledge to reasonably prescribe exercise as a means of maintaining or improving cognitive performance. In this review, the first step was to examine large-scale prospective studies in which physical activity levels were adequately quantified and to examine changes in cognitive performance over time as a function of activity level. The second step was to review the findings of meta-analytic reviews in which the factors that define the dose of physical activity were examined as potential moderators of cognitive effect size. The third step was to review the literature with respect to the underlying mediators and mechanisms (intervening variables) that have been proposed to explain a link between physical activity and cognition. If dose–response relationships have been observed between these underlying variables and cognitive performance, physical activity prescription could be informed by the dose–response relationship between physical activity and these intervening variables with an ultimate goal of affecting cognitive performance.

Prospective Studies

Several groups of researchers have used large-scale prospective designs to study the relationship between physical activity and cognitive performance over time. All of these studies have been conducted with older adults; thus results may not generalize to other age groups. The results of these studies have been mixed; this is undoubtedly related to the variety of cognitive outcomes and physical activity measures that have been used and the differences in the amount of time between measurements. One group of studies has focused on performance on standardized cognitive measures as the outcome, and another group has focused on the assessment of clinical cognitive impairments as the outcome. The specific method of assessing physical activity in these studies has varied, but has been limited to self-report measures.

Physical Activity and Cognitive Performance

Four prospective studies have been conducted in which a measure of physical activity was tested as a predictor of cognitive performance at a subsequent testing time or as a predictor of the change in cognitive performance over time.

Albert and colleagues (1995) reported findings from 1119 participants (70-79 years) in the MacArthur Studies of Successful Aging. Physical activity (assessed as current level of participation in strenuous physical activities) was used to predict change in performance on a battery of cognitive tests over a five-year period. Using structural equation modeling, physical activity was found to be a significant predictor of cognitive change such that higher levels of strenuous physical activity were predictive of less cognitive decline over time.

Dik and colleagues (2003) assessed physical activity and cognitive performance in 1241 older adults (62-85 years). They assessed early-life physical activity behavior retrospectively at baseline by asking participants to report how many hours per week they participated in sport or other physical activity when they were 15 to 25 years of age. Cognitive performance was then assessed over a six-year follow-up period. Results showed that performance on the Mini-Mental State Exam (MMSE) and information-processing speed were predicted by physical activity such that low or moderate early-life physical activity was predictive of significantly better performance than no early-life physical activity.

Van Gelder and colleagues (2004) measured the frequency, duration, and intensity of physical activity of 295 older men ($M = 74.91$ years) taking part in the Finland, Italy, and The Netherlands Elderly (FINE) Study. Physical activity change was operationalized as decreasing, remaining stable, or increasing in duration and intensity over a 10-year period. Results demonstrated that change in duration and change in intensity of physical activity participation were predictive of cognitive decline on the MMSE in a dose–response pattern, with increasing duration and intensity of physical activity predictive of less decline in cognitive performance (see table 9.1).

Weuve and colleagues (2004) assessed physical activity in 16,466 older women (70-81 years) at two-year intervals for 10 to 17 years prior to the measurement of cognitive performance. They assessed physical activity by asking participants to estimate the average amount of time per week spent performing a variety of aerobic activities and other low-intensity physical activities (e.g., yoga). The data were converted into metabolic equivalents (METs) and averaged over the time period prior to the cognitive assessment. Results indicated that physical activity was predictive of better cognitive performance, with the pattern of results across quintiles of physical activity demonstrating a dose–response relationship such that increasing levels of physical activity were associated with better cognitive performance (see table 9.2).

Physical Activity and Clinical Cognitive Impairment

Seven large-scale prospective studies have been conducted in which baseline physical activity was assessed and the incidence of clinical cognitive impairment was then measured after a number of years.

Yaffe and colleagues (2001) explored the relationship between baseline physical activity and cognitive change on the MMSE over six to eight years

Table 9.1 **Mean Change in MMSE Performance Over 10 Years Relative to the Change in Duration and Intensity of Physical Activity**

	Decrease in PA	No change in PA	Increase in PA
Duration	−1.7	−0.7	0.0
Intensity	−2.3	−0.6	0.2

Note: PA = physical activity.

Data from B.M. Gelder et al., 2004, "Physical activity in relation to cognitive decline in elderly men: The FINE Study," *Neurology, 63*(12), 2316-2321.

in 5925 older women (>65 years). Physical activity was assessed as self-reported blocks of walking per week and the frequency and duration of participation in 33 different types of physical activity (converted to kilocalories). Results for blocks walked per week and for kilocalories supported a dose–response relationship, with an increase in activity being associated with less risk of clinical cognitive decline (see table 9.3).

Laurin and colleagues (2001) presented data from the Canadian Study of Health and Aging. Older adults (>65 years, $n = 4615$) without dementia self-reported their physical activity at baseline and were then tested for

Table 9.2   Mean Differences in Cognitive Performance Relative to Physical Activity Quintile

Outcome measure	Physical activity quintile				
	Lowest	2nd lowest	Middle	2nd highest	Highest
TICS	0.0 (Ref)	0.20	0.27	0.28	0.28
Category fluency	0.0 (Ref)	0.59	0.74	0.76	0.95
Working memory and attention	0.0 (Ref)	0.15	0.16	0.27	0.34
Verbal memory	0.0 (Ref)	0.04	0.03	0.07	0.08
Global score	0.0 (Ref)	0.06	0.06	0.09	0.10

Note: TICS = telephone interview for cognitive status (modeled after the Mini-Mental State Exam); Ref = referent group.

Data from J. Weuve et al., 2004, "Physical activity, including walking, and cognitive function in older women," *Journal of the American Medical Association* 292(12), 1454-1461.

Table 9.3   Odds Ratios for Cognitive Decline Relative to Physical Activity

Physical activity measure	Physical activity quartile			
	Lowest	2nd lowest	2nd highest	Highest
Blocks walked	1.0 (Ref)	0.87	0.63	0.66
kcal	1.0 (Ref)	0.90	0.78	0.74

Note: Ref = referent group.

Data from K. Yaffe et al., 2001, "A prospective study of physical activity and cognitive decline in elderly women—Women who walk," *Archives of Internal Medicine* 161(14), 1703-1708.

clinical cognitive impairment at a five-year follow-up. Physical activity was reported as the frequency (number of times per week) and the intensity of exercise, which were combined into a single composite score with four levels (high, moderate, low, none). Results supported a dose–response relationship, with higher levels of physical activity participation generally being predictive of a lesser risk of clinical cognitive impairment (see table 9.4).

Wilson and colleagues (2002) reported findings from the Chicago Health and Aging Project. In this study, self-report measures of physical activity were assessed in 835 older adults (>65 years) and then, after an average of 4.1 years, incident Alzheimer's disease was ascertained. The researchers assessed physical activity by asking participants how often and for how long they had performed any of nine physical activities over the past two weeks. Results indicated that physical activity participation was not predictive of the risk of Alzheimer's disease.

Verghese and coworkers (2003) reported findings from the Bronx Aging Study, in which self-report measures of baseline physical activity (11 activities provided) and the frequency of participation in these activities were assessed in 488 older adults (75-85 years). Incident dementia was then assessed over a median time period of 5.1 years (maximum = 21 years). Results demonstrated that physical activity was not associated with the risk of Alzheimer's disease.

In another study, Abbott and colleagues (2004) asked 2257 relatively healthy older men (71-93 years) to self-report the average number of miles walked per day and then followed the participants for an average of seven years to determine incident dementia. Results supported a dose–response

Table 9.4   Odds Ratios for Risk of Cognitive Impairment Relative to Physical Activity Level

	Physical activity level			
Outcome measure	None	Low	Moderate	High
Cognitive impairment (not dementia)	1.00 (Ref)	0.66	0.67	0.58
Alzheimer's disease	1.00 (Ref)	0.67	0.67	0.50
Vascular dementia	1.00 (Ref)	0.54	0.70	0.63
Any type of dementia	1.00 (Ref)	0.64	0.69	0.63

Note: Ref = referent group.

Data from D. Laurin et al., 2001, "Physical activity and risk of cognitive impairment and dementia in elderly persons," *Archives of Neurology* 53(3): 498-504.

relationship between walking and cognitive function; the relative hazard of dementia increased with decreased distance walked (>2 miles: referent; >1 to 2 miles: 1.50; 0.25 to 1 miles: 2.06; ≤0.25 miles: 2.12).

As previously described, Weuve and colleagues (2004) used the average volume of physical activity over an 8- to 15-year period to predict cognitive performance in 16,466 older women. Results indicated that women in the highest quintile for physical activity participation were at 20% lower risk of cognitive impairment than women in the lowest quintile.

Podewils and colleagues (2005) examined the relationship between physical activity and the development of dementia over a period of 5.4 years in older adults (>65 years). Physical activity was self-reported as the frequency and duration of participation in 15 physical activities over the previous two weeks. Although the effects were not all statistically significant, results consistently demonstrated a dose–response relationship for risk of clinical cognitive impairment with both energy expenditure (calculated from frequency and duration) and the number of different physical activities (see table 9.5). The general thrust of the results was that increasing energy expenditure and an increasing variety of activities were predictive of less risk of clinical impairment.

Table 9.5   Crude Hazard Ratios for Risk of Clinical Cognitive Impairment Relative to Physical Activity

Clinical impairment	Energy expenditure (kcal/week)			
	<248	248-742	743-1657	>1657
All-cause dementia	1.0 (Ref)	1.03	0.81	0.74
Alzheimer's disease	1.0 (Ref)	0.99	0.79	0.64
Vascular dementia	1.0 (Ref)	1.04	0.90	0.82
Clinical impairment	Number of physical activities			
	0-1	2	3	≥4
All-cause dementia	1.0 (Ref)	0.76	0.60	0.42
Alzheimer's disease	1.0 (Ref)	0.68	0.61	0.40
Vascular dementia	1.0 (Ref)	0.85	0.64	0.44

Note: Ref = referent group.

Data from L.J. Podewils et al., 2005, "Physical activity, APOE genotype, and dementia risk: findings from the Cardiovascular Health Cognition Study," *American Journal of Epidemiology* 161(7): 639-651.

The results of these large-scale prospective studies have been generally consistent with support for a dose–response relationship provided by all of the studies of cognitive performance outcomes and by five of the seven studies that used clinical cognitive impairment as the outcome variable. An examination of the two studies that failed to support the relationship indicates that these two studies used a relatively short follow-up period (see table 9.6) and did not include an indication of intensity of physical activity. Thus, from this line of evidence it can be concluded that a dose–response relationship between physical activity and cognitive performance exists in

Table 9.6   **Descriptive Information for Prospective Studies Examining the Relationship Between Physical Activity and Cognitive Performance or the Experience of Clinical Cognitive Impairment**

Authors (year)	Sex	Age	Follow-up measure (years)	Physical activity measure
Cognitive performance supporting (4 of 4)				
Albert et al. (1995)	M, F	70-79	5	Strenuous activity
Dik et al. (2003)	M	62-85	6	Early-life physical activity
van Gelder et al. (2004)	M, F	74.91	10	Change in duration and intensity
Weuve et al. (2004)	F	70-81	10-17	Time per week and type → METs
Clinical impairment supporting (5 of 7)				
Yaffe et al. (2001)	F	>65	6-8	Blocks walked, kcal
Laurin et al. (2001)	M, F	>65	5	Frequency and intensity
Abbott et al. (2004)	M	71-93	7	Number of miles walked per day
Weuve et al. (2004)	F	70-81	10-17	Time per week and type → METs
Podewils et al. (2005)	M, F	>65	5.4	Frequency, duration, type → kcal
Clinical impairment failing to support (2 of 7)				
Wilson et al. (2002)	M, F	>65	4.1	Frequency and duration
Verghese et al. (2003)	M, F	75-85	5.1	Type and frequency

Note: M = males, F = females, METs = metabolic equivalents, kcal = kilocalories.

older adults, that "more is better" and that physical activity intensity is an important component of the dose of physical activity.

Meta-Analytic Reviews

Several meta-analytic reviews have been conducted to statistically summarize the relationship between physical activity and cognitive performance. These meta-analyses have often explored the impact of moderator variables on the relationship and therefore provide a statistical test of the various aspects of physical activity that might be predictive of cognitive performance.

Etnier and colleagues (1997) statistically reviewed 46 long-term exercise studies with people of all ages (4-94 years) in which an exercise intervention was implemented and cognitive performance was measured at the posttest (and compared either to a pretest score or to a control group's posttest score). Effect sizes (ES) were calculated for the cognitive measure, and then moderators related to the dose of the exercise intervention were statistically examined to determine their influence on the cognitive ES. The average ES for these studies was 0.33, supporting a small effect of exercise on cognitive performance. However, when the moderator variables were analyzed, results indicated that neither mode (aerobic, muscular resistance, games, other), intensity (low, moderate, high), duration (1-180 min), frequency (two to seven days per week), nor length of the physical activity program (3-42 weeks) significantly influenced the size of the cognitive ES ($p > .05$). Thus, the authors concluded that although there was evidence to support a causal link between physical activity and cognitive performance, there was no evidence to support a dose–response relationship between these variables. The findings from this meta-analytic review suggest that the prescription of physical activity to benefit cognitive performance does not need to specify anything other than a general increase in physical activity level.

Sibley and Etnier (2003) meta-analytically reviewed 44 studies in which physical activity and cognition were examined in children. Their overall results also supported a small effect of physical activity on cognitive performance ($ES = 0.32$). The authors analyzed these effects relative to mode of exercise (resistance or circuit training, physical education class, aerobic exercise, perceptual-motor training) and found that this moderator did not significantly affect the findings. This suggests that, for children, the prescription of physical activity to improve cognitive performance does not need to specify a particular type of activity.

Colcombe and Kramer (2003) conducted a meta-analytic review that included only studies involving older adults (55-80 years) and using experimental designs. Their overall findings demonstrated a moderate ES ($ES = 0.48$). Colcombe and Kramer then examined these effects relative to duration and mode of sessions and the length of the exercise intervention (see table 9.7). With regard to the duration of sessions, findings indicated that sessions of moderate duration (31-45 min) had a significantly larger average effect than did interventions using long duration (46-60 min) or short duration (15-30 min), and also that long-duration sessions were significantly more effective than sessions of short duration. With respect to the mode of exercise, results demonstrated significantly larger effects with a combined program of strength training and aerobic training than with aerobic training administered alone. Finally, findings for program length showed significantly larger effects for long programs (more than six months) than for short programs (one to three months) or moderate-length programs (four to six months) and demonstrated that short programs had bigger effects than moderate-length programs. These results suggest that the dose of the physical activity intervention influences the magnitude of the cognitive ES, but also indicate that this relationship is not linear. This counterintuitive finding may be a result of the limitations inherent in meta-analytic reviews (to be discussed below). However, based on the results of this meta-analysis, the prescription of physical activity to improve cognitive performance in older adults would suggest the adoption of interventions with 31 to 45 min of aerobic and strength training for more than six months.

Before discussing of the overall conclusions that can be drawn from these meta-analytic reviews, the limitations of the reviews must be understood. One limitation is that findings from meta-analytic reviews are, by defini-

Table 9.7   Effect Sizes Relative to the Dose–Response Moderators From the Colcombe and Kramer (2003) Meta-Analysis

	15-30 min	31-45 min	45-60 min
Duration	0.18[b2]	0.61[a]	0.47[b1]

	Aerobic only	Strength and aerobic	
Mode	0.41[b]	0.59[a]	

	1-3 months	4-6 months	>6 months
Length of program	0.52[b1]	0.27[b2]	0.67[a]

Note: Superscripts indicate which levels of the moderator are significantly different from one another. Effects that have different numbers are significantly different from one another, and effects that have different letters are significantly different from one another.

Data from S. Colcombe and A.F. Kramer, 2003, "Fitness effects on the cognitive function of older adults: A meta-analytic study," *Psychological Science* 14(2): 125-130.

tion, the result of statistically summarizing the extant literature and do not necessarily represent the findings that would result from any single study. In other words, the analyses with respect to the moderator variables are limited by the particular manner in which the ES "fall out" relative to the levels of the moderator variables. One way in which this can affect the findings occurs when there are small numbers of studies in the various levels of the moderator variables. As an example, in Etnier and colleagues' (1997) meta-analysis, the number of studies that used anaerobic interventions (n = 3) and the number of studies that used high-intensity exercise (n = 2) were extremely small. Thus, the statistical power for the relevant moderator variables was low, and as a result, meaningful differences in ES as a function of these variables might not have reached statistical significance. A second way in which the findings of a meta-analysis are affected involves a phenomenon referred to as third-order causation. This occurs when two (or more) moderator variables overlap with one another so that the individual effect of either on the outcome variable is confounded by the other. As an example, in the Colcombe and Kramer meta-analysis (2003), the largest cognitive ES were observed for studies in which executive function tasks were used to assess cognitive performance. It is possible that findings with regard to the dose–response moderators might have been confounded by this moderator variable. That is, perhaps the studies that contributed ES to the moderate-duration (31-45 min) sessions were also those that assessed executive function tasks. This would cause the moderate-duration sessions to demonstrate a large average effect, but the effect might be more reflective of the cognitive task that was used than of the duration of the sessions. Third-order causation could also influence findings in the reverse direction. That is, perhaps the dose–response moderators in Etnier and coworkers' (1997) meta-analysis did not demonstrate significant effects because they overlapped with another moderator variable in a way that dampened the effects. This is a limitation inherent in all meta-analyses and must be kept in mind as the findings of meta-analyses are interpreted. The only way to address this limitation is to examine the effects of the moderators in a single study; however, to my knowledge there is no published study in which parameters that define the dose of the exercise intervention have been manipulated to directly investigate this relationship.

Taken as a whole, the results of the meta-analytic reviews of the literature suggest that in the general population and in children, a dose–response relationship has not been demonstrated but that one can expect any increase in physical activity to be associated with an improvement in cognitive performance. However, in older adults, there is support for a dose–response relationship, and the meta-analytic results suggest that this relationship is not linear. In particular, the findings from the Colcombe and Kramer (2003) meta-analysis indicate that the largest effects are evident for short (one to three months) and long (more than six months) interventions, for sessions that are moderate (31-45 min) in length, and for physical activity that includes both strength training and aerobic components.

Mediators and Mechanisms

A third way of evaluating the evidence relative to a prescription of exercise is to consider the dose–response literature in relation to mediators and mechanisms that are thought to underlie the observed relationship between physical activity and cognitive performance. Potential mediators of the relationship that have been suggested include aerobic fitness, depression, sleep quality, anxiety, and self-efficacy. Potential biological mechanisms that have been proposed include cerebral structure, cerebral metabolism, neurotransmitters, neurotrophic factors, oxygen availability, glucose regulation, and oxidative stress. Unfortunately, while this approach to evaluating the literature would provide valuable indirect evidence regarding dose–response relationships, this process is critically limited by the lack of research in which mediators and mechanisms (intervening variables) have been appropriately tested. That is, these intervening variables have typically been examined in a piecemeal fashion, with studies focusing on the relationship between physical activity and the proposed intervening variable or between the proposed intervening variable and cognitive performance. To my knowledge, there is no study with humans in which physical activity has been manipulated, intervening variables have been measured, and the effects of these intervening variables on cognitive performance have been statistically tested (see Etnier, 2008).

The only intervening variable that has been studied to any extent from a dose–response perspective is aerobic fitness. This is likely reflective of the physiological link between physical activity and aerobic fitness and the popularity of the cardiovascular fitness hypothesis, which suggests that the mental health benefits of physical activity are due to the responses of the cardiovascular system to the metabolic demands of regular physical activity (Barnes, Yaffe, Satariano, & Tager, 2003). Should the evidence support a dose–response relationship between aerobic fitness and cognitive performance, then, given the wealth of knowledge regarding the dose of physical activity needed to produce a specific gain in aerobic fitness, this information could guide the design of a physical activity intervention that would produce the appropriate gain in aerobic fitness and have the desired effect on cognitive performance.

In order to evaluate the literature to determine if there is, in fact, a dose–response relationship between aerobic fitness and cognitive performance, three steps were taken. First, empirical studies using chronic exercise paradigms were reviewed to identify the initial level of aerobic fitness, the change in aerobic fitness (absolute and relative), and whether or not the results demonstrated an effect on cognitive performance. The evidence from these studies is mixed, with 15 studies demonstrating a causal relationship between aerobic fitness and cognitive performance and 7 studies failing to support this relationship. Examination of the data (see table 9.8) demonstrates that the range of relative change in aerobic fitness is broad and similar for the 15 studies that supported (1-27% gain) and the 7 studies that failed to support (12-23% gain) an effect. Thus, examination of the empirical studies aimed at testing the causal relationship between aerobic fitness and cognitive performance provides mixed support for a causal link and does not support a dose–response relationship between these variables.

Second, results from meta-analytic reviews that specifically tested aerobic fitness gains as a moderator of the relationship between physical activity and cognitive performance were examined. Etnier and colleagues (1997) found no significant differences in ES as a function of whether or not significant gains in aerobic fitness were reported by the authors of the studies reviewed. Similarly, Colcombe and Kramer (2003) reported that there were no significant differences in ES as a function of categories of improvement in aerobic fitness (unreported, 5-11% gain, 12-25% gain). These findings suggest that there is not a dose–response relationship between aerobic fitness and cognitive performance.

Third, Etnier and colleagues (2006) conducted a meta-analytic review designed to test the mediating role of aerobic fitness in the relationship between physical activity and cognitive performance. Meta-regression techniques were used to test the ability of the change in aerobic fitness to predict the change in cognitive performance using data from 37 studies. Results indicated that change in aerobic fitness was not predictive of change in cognitive performance.

Overall, the results of narrative and meta-analytic reviews fail to support a dose–response relationship between aerobic fitness and cognitive performance. However, as mentioned previously, these conclusions are constrained by the designs of the existing studies, by third-order causation, and by the fact that there has not been a large-scale RCT in which aerobic fitness has been systematically manipulated so that the dose–response relationship with cognitive performance can be tested.

One large-scale prospective study tested the dose–response relationship between aerobic fitness and cognitive performance. Barnes and colleagues (2003) examined the relationship between aerobic fitness (peak $\dot{V}O_2$) and cognitive change on the MMSE over a six-year period in 349 older adults (>55 years). Results indicated that baseline aerobic fitness was predictive of MMSE change scores, with the amount of decline decreasing with increasing levels of aerobic fitness (lowest fitness: –0.5; middle fitness: –0.2; highest fitness: 0.0). Similar patterns of results were observed with other cognitive tests that were administered (Trails B, Stroop, Digit Symbol, Immediate Recall, Delayed Recall on the California Verbal Learning Tool,

171

Table 9.8   **Published Studies in Which Physical Activity Was Manipulated**

Study	$\dot{V}O_2$ change (ml · kg^{-1} · min^{-1})	Pretest $\dot{V}O_2$max (ml · kg^{-1} · min^{-1})	% change pretest to posttest	Age range and/or (average age)
		Supporting (n = 15)		
Kramer et al. (2002)	0.30	21.5	1%	60-75
Emery et al. (2003)	0.51	14.64	3%	>50
Etnier & Berry (2001)	0.94	18.27	5%	55-80
Harma et al. (1988)	1.90	33.20	6%	(35.00)
Hascelik et al. (1989)	3.35	37.20	9%	17-20 (18.50)
Zervas et al. (1991)	5.42	52.07	10%	11-14 (13.10)
Colcombe et al. (2004)	nr	nr	10%	58-77 (65.60)
Hassmen et al. (1992)	3	27.4	11%	55-75
Khatri et al. (2001)	2.79	20.22	14%	50-72 (56.73)
Emery et al. (1998)	2.00	12.40	16%	>50 (65.4)
Ismail & El-Naggar (1981)	8.30	43.70	19%	24-68 (42.00)
El-Naggar (1986)	6.58	35.23	19%	25-65
Moul et al. (1995)	4.20	22.4	19%	65-72 (69.1)
Blomquist & Danner (1987)	8.10	34.70	23%	18-48 (28.10)
Dustman et al. (1984)	5.20	19.4	27%	55-68 (61.00)
Range	0.30 – 8.30	12.40-52.07	1-27%	

Study	$\dot{V}O_2$ change (ml · kg⁻¹ · min⁻¹)	Pretest $\dot{V}O_2$max (ml · kg⁻¹ · min⁻¹)	% change pretest to posttest	Age range and/or (average age)
Failing to support (n = 7)				
Madden et al. (1989)	2.27	19.69	12%	60-83 (66.00)
Blumenthal & Madden (1988)	5.35	34.54	15%	30-58 (43.32)
Whitehurst (1991)	4.20	25.48	16%	61-73 (65.80)
Pierce et al. (1993)	5.09	31.8	16%	29-59 (44.30)
Blaney et al. (1990)	8	45	18%	(42.00)
Panton et al. (1990)	4.6	22.5	20%	70-79 (71.92)
Hill et al. (1993)	5.52	24.53	23%	60-73 (64.00)
Range	2.27–8.00	19.69-34.54	12-23%	

Note: In all these studies, changes in aerobic fitness were reported as ml · kg⁻¹ · min⁻¹, and changes in cognitive performance were reported as either supporting or failing to support a positive effect.

verbal fluency). These results demonstrate that when examined in a single study using a prospective design, a dose–response relationship between aerobic fitness and cognitive performance can be observed.

A review of the evidence using mediators and mechanisms to inform dose–response questions related to physical activity and cognition is limited to a focus on aerobic fitness. Results with aerobic fitness generally suggest that the amount of change in fitness is not predictive of the amount of change in cognitive performance. The one exception is that findings from a prospective study (Barnes et al., 2003) with older adults do support a dose–response relationship, with higher levels of aerobic fitness being predictive of less cognitive decline over a six-year period.

Conclusions

The question driving this review was whether or not the existing evidence is such that we are ready to prescribe physical activity (mode, intensity, duration, frequency) to improve or protect cognitive functioning. The evidence that has been reviewed generally supports a positive relationship between physical activity and cognitive performance; however, the evidence regarding the dose–response relationship between physical activity and cognitive performance is less clear, and the conclusions that can be drawn from this review are different for children and adults than for older adults.

This review clearly demonstrates that there is a paucity of research on the dose–response relationship between physical activity and cognitive performance in the general population and in children. Given that meta-analytic reviews consistently support a small positive relationship between physical activity and cognition in children and in adults, future research is needed in which dose–response relationships are specifically examined in these populations. At this point, we are not ready to do more than generally prescribe an increase in physical activity to promote cognitive performance in children and in the general population.

Substantially more studies on this relationship have been conducted with older adults. A review of this literature generally supports the existence of a dose–response relationship between physical activity and cognitive performance for older adults, although the specific nature of this relationship requires clarification. Large-scale prospective studies with older adults suggest that higher levels of energy expenditure (Abbott et al., 2004; Albert et al., 1995; Dik et al., 2003; Laurin et al., 2001; Podewils et al., 2005; van Gelder et al., 2004; Weuve et al., 2004; Yaffe et al., 2001) and higher levels of aerobic fitness (Barnes et al., 2003) are predictive of better cognitive performance and less cognitive decline over time. In contrast, a meta-analytic review of experimental studies with older adults (Colcombe & Kramer, 2003) suggests that a moderate duration of exercise produces significantly larger effects than do shorter or longer durations, and that the evidence does not support a dose–response relationship between aerobic fitness and cognitive performance. Thus, in general with older adults, the results support a dose–response relationship; but they seem to suggest that while higher levels of energy expenditure and of aerobic fitness are associated with larger cognitive effects over a period of several years, physical activity does not need to be performed at a level that results in improvements in cardiovascular fitness in order for these benefits to be observed in the short term.

Given the lack of systematic study of these relationships from a dose–response perspective, I strongly encourage future researchers to use the evidence from the prospective literature to support the design of RCTs in which physical activity is manipulated in a dose–response fashion and effects on cognition are assessed.

Summary

At this point, the prescription of physical activity for the protection or improvement of cognitive performance is warranted, but the specifics of the prescription have not been clarified. Given that physical health benefits are expected to accrue when physical activity is performed according to the recommendations of the ACSM and the CDC, as well as the fact that these recommendations do not conflict with the findings of this review, it seems practical at this point to recommend a combination of aerobic and strength training for 20 to 60 min on all or most days of the week and to caution that a commitment of six months or longer may be necessary for cognitive effects to become evident. Future research is needed before more specific cognitive-enhancing physical activity prescriptions can be offered.

Chapter 1

Alain, C., & Woods, D.L. (1999). Age-related changes in processing auditory stimuli during visual attention: evidence for deficits in inhibitory control and sensory memory. *Psychology and Aging, 14*, 507-519.

Birren, J.E., & Fisher, L.M. (1995). Aging and speed of behavior: possible consequences for psychological functioning. *Annual Review of Psychology, 46*, 329-353.

Bowles, R.P., & Salthouse, T.A. (2003). Assessing the age-related effects of proactive interference on working memory tasks using the Rasch model. *Psychology and Aging, 18*, 608-615.

Brumback, C., Gratton, G., & Fabiani, M. (2005a). Working memory capacity differences in older and younger adults. *Journal of Cognitive Neuroscience Supplement*, p. 101.

Brumback, C.R., Low, K., Gratton, G., & Fabiani, M. (2005b). Putting things into perspective: differences in working memory span and the integration of information. *Experimental Psychology, 52*, 21-30.

Cabeza, R. (2002). Hemispheric asymmetry reduction in older adults: the HAROLD model. *Psychology and Aging, 17*, 85-100.

Cabeza, R., Grady, C.L., Nyberg, L., McIntosh, A.R., Tulving, E., Kapur, S., Jennings, J.M., Houle, S., & Craik, F.I. (1997). Age-related differences in neural activity during memory encoding and retrieval: a positron emission tomography study. *Journal of Neuroscience, 17*, 391-400.

Colcombe, S.J., Kramer, A.F., Erickson, K.I., & Scalp, P. (2005). The implications of cortical recruitment and brain morphology in cognitive performance in aging in humans. *Psychology and Aging, 20*(3), 363-375.

Craik, F.I.M., & Byrd, M. (1982). Aging and cognitive deficits: the role of attentional resources. In F.I.M. Craik & S. Trehub (Eds.), *Aging and cognitive processes* (pp. 191-211). New York: Plenum Press.

Czigler, I., Csibra, G., & Csontos, A. (1992). Age and inter-stimulus interval effects on event-related potentials to frequent and infrequent auditory stimuli. *Biological Psychology, 33*(2-3), 195-206.

Donchin, E. (1981). Surprise! . . . surprise? *Psychophysiology, 18*, 493-513.

Donchin, E., & Coles, M.G.H. (1988). Is the P300 component a manifestation of context updating? *Behavioral and Brain Sciences, 11*, 355-372.

Fabiani, M., Brumback, C., Gordon, B., Pearson, M., Lee, Y., Kramer, A., McAuley, E., & Gratton, G. (2004a). Effects of cardiopulmonary fitness on neurovascular coupling in visual cortex in younger and older adults. *Psychophysiology, 41*, S19.

Fabiani, M., Brumback, C.R., Pearson, M.A., Gordon, B.A., Lee, Y., Barre, M., O'Dell, J., Maclin, E.L., Elavsky, S. Konopack, J.F., McAuley, E., Kramer, A.F., & Gratton, G. (2005). Neurovascular coupling in young and old adults assessed with neuronal (EROS) and hemodynamic (NIRS) optical imaging measures. *Journal of Cognitive Neuroscience Supplement, 34.*

Fabiani, M., & Friedman, D. (1995). Changes in brain activity patterns in aging: the novelty oddball. *Psychophysiology, 32*, 579-594.

Fabiani, M., Gratton, G., Corballis, P., Cheng, J., & Friedman, D. (1998). Bootstrap assessment of the reliability of maxima in surface maps of brain activity of individual subjects derived with electrophysiological and optical methods. *Behavior Research Methods, Instruments, and Computers, 30*, 78-86.

Fabiani, M., Gratton, G., & Federmeier, K. (2007). Event-related brain potentials. In J. Cacioppo, L. Tassinary, & G. Berntson (Eds.), *Handbook of Psychophysiology* (3rd Edition) (pp. 85-119). New York: Cambridge University Press.

Fabiani, M., Low, K.A., Wee, E., Sable, J.J., & Gratton, G. (2006). Reduced suppression or labile memory? Mechanisms of inefficient filtering of irrelevant information in older adults. *Journal of Cognitive Neuroscience, 18(4)*, 637-650.

Fox, P.T., & Raichle, M.E. (1985). Stimulus rate determines regional brain blood flow in striate cortex. *Annals of Neurology, 17*, 303-305.

Gaeta, H., Friedman, D., Ritter, W., & Cheng, J. (1998). An event-related potential study of age-related changes in sensitivity to stimulus deviance. *Neurobiology of Aging, 19*(5), 447-459.

Golob, E.J., Miranda, G.G., Johnson, J.K., & Starr, A. (2001). Sensory cortical interactions in aging, mild cognitive impairment, and Alzheimer's disease. *Neurobiology of Aging, 22*, 755-763.

Gordon, B., Rykhlevskaia, E. Brumback, C.R., Lee, Y., Elavsky, S., Konopack, J.F., McAuley, E., Kramer, A.F., Colcombe, S., Gratton, G., & Fabiani, M. (2008). Anotomical correlates of aging, cardiopulmonary fitness level, and education. *Psychophysiology, 45(5)*, 825-838.

Gratton, G., Corballis, P.M., Cho, E., Fabiani, M., & Hood, D. (1995). Shades of gray matter: noninvasive optical images of human brain responses during visual stimulation. *Psychophysiology, 32*, 505-509.

Gratton, G., & Fabiani, M. (2001). Shedding light on brain function: the event-related optical signal. *Trends in Cognitive Sciences, 5*, 357-363.

Gratton, G., & Fabiani, M. (2003). The event related optical signal (EROS) in visual cortex: replicability, consistency, localization and resolution. *Psychophysiology, 40*, 561-571.

References

Gratton, G., Goodman-Wood, M.R., & Fabiani, M. (2001). Comparison of neuronal and hemodynamic measures of the brain response to visual stimulation: an optical imaging study. *Human Brain Mapping, 13(1),* 13-25.

Gratton, G., Rykhlevskaia, E. Wee, E., Leaver, E., & Fabiani, M. (in press). Does white matter matter? Spatiotemporal dynamics of task switching in aging. *Journal of Cognitive Neuroscience.*

Hasher, L., & Zacks, R.T. (1988). Working memory, comprehension, and aging: a review and a new view. In G.H. Bower (Ed.), *The psychology of learning and motivation* (Vol. 22, pp. 193-225). New York: Academic Press.

Kane, M.J., & Engle, R.W. (2000). Working-memory capacity, proactive interference, and divided attention: limits on long-term memory retrieval. *Journal of Experimental Psychology: Learning, Memory, and Cognition, 26,* 336-358.

Kausler, D.H., & Hakami, M.K. (1982). Frequency judgments by young and elderly adults for relevant stimuli with simultaneously present irrelevant stimuli. *Journal of Gerontology, 37,* 438-442.

Kazmerski, V.A., Friedman, D., & Ritter, W. (1997). Mismatch negativity during attend and ignore conditions in Alzheimer's disease. *Biological Psychiatry, 42*(5), 382-402.

Kazmerski, V.A., Lee, Y., Gratton, G., and Fabiani, M. (2005). Evidence for inefficient sensory filtering mechanisms in aging. *Journal of Cognitive Neuroscience Supplement, 89-90.*

Klein, M., Coles, M.G.H., & Donchin, E. (1984). People with absolute pitch process tones without producing a P300. *Science, 223,* 1306-1309.

Knight, R.T. (1984). Decreased response to novel stimuli after prefrontal lesions in man. *Electroencephalography and Clinical Neurophysiology, 59,* 9-20.

Knight, R.T., & Grabowecky, M. (1995). Escape from linear time: prefrontal cortex and conscious experience. In M. Gazzaniga (Ed.), *The cognitive neurosciences* (pp. 1357-1371). Cambridge: MIT Press.

Knight, R.T., Hillyard, S.A., Woods, D.L., & Neville, H.J. (1980). The effects of frontal and temporal-parietal lesions on the auditory evoked potential in man. *Electroencephalography and Clinical Neurophysiology, 50,* 112-124.

Moscovitch, M., & Winocur, G. (1992). The neuropsychology of memory and aging. In F.I.M. Craik & T.A. Salthouse (Eds.), *The handbook of aging and cognition* (pp. 315-372). Hillsdale, NJ: Erlbaum.

Park, D.C., Smith, A.D., Lautenschlager, G., Earles, J., Frieske, D., Zwahr, M., & Gaines, C. (1996). Mediators of long-term memory performance across the life span. *Psychology and Aging, 11,* 621-637.

Pekkonen, E. Rinne, T. Reinikainen, K., Kujala, T., Alho, K., & Näätänen, R. (1996). Aging effects on auditory processing: an event-related potential study. *Experimental Aging Research, 22*(2), 171-184.

Polich, J., Howard, L., & Starr, A. (1985). Effects of age on the P300 component of the event-related potential from auditory stimuli: peak definition, variation, and measurement. *Journal of Gerontology, 40,* 721-726.

Rabbitt, P. (1965). Age-decrement in the ability to ignore irrelevant information. *Journal of Gerontology, 20,* 233-238.

Reuter-Lorenz, P.A., Jonides, J., Smith, E.E., Hartley, A., Miller, A., Marshuetz, C., & Koeppe, R.A. (2000). Age differences in the frontal lateralization of verbal and spatial working memory revealed by PET. *Journal of Cognitive Neuroscience, 12,* 174-187.

Ritter, W., Deacon, D., Gomes, H., Javitt, D.C., & Vaughan, H.G., Jr. (1995). The mismatch negativity of event-related potentials as a probe of transient auditory memory: a review. *Ear and Hearing, 16,* 52-67.

Sable, J.J., Low, K.A., Maclin, E.L., Fabiani, M., & Gratton, G. (2004). Latent inhibition mediates N1 attenuation to repeating sounds. *Psychophysiology, 41,* 636-642.

Sable, J.J., Wee, E., Low, K.A., Gratton, G, & Fabiani, M. (in preparation). Increased involuntary attention, but not faster decay of sensory memory with age.

Salthouse, T.A. (1996). The processing-speed theory of adult age differences in cognition. *Psychological Review, 103*(3), 403-428.

Smulders, F.T., Kenemans, J.L., Schmidt, W.F., & Kok, A. (1999). Effects of task complexity in young and old adults: reaction time and P300 latency are not always dissociated. *Psychophysiology, 36,* 118-125.

Squires, K., Petuchowski, S., Wickens, C., & Donchin, E. (1977). The effects of stimulus sequence on event related potentials: a comparison of visual and auditory sequences. *Perception and Psychophysics, 22,* 31-40.

Sutton, S., Braren, M., Zubin, J., & John, E.R. (1965). Evoked-potential correlates of stimulus uncertainty. *Science, 150,* 1187-1188.

Villringer, A., & Chance, B. (1997). Non-invasive optical spectroscopy and imaging of human brain function. *Trends in Neuroscience, 20,* 435-442.

Villringer, A., & Dirnagl, U. (1995). Coupling of brain activity and cerebral blood flow: basis of functional neuroimaging. *Cerebrovascular and Brain Metabolism Reviews, 7,* 240-276.

West, R.L. (1996). An application of prefrontal cortex function theory to cognitive aging. *Psychological Bulletin, 120*(2), 272-292.

Woodruff-Pak, D.S. (1997). *The neuropsychology of aging* (Vol. 352). Cambridge, MA: Blackwell.

Woods, D.L. (1992). Auditory selective attention in middle-aged and elderly subjects: an event-related brain potential study. *Electroencephalography and Clinical Neurophysiology, 84*(5), 456-468.

Yamaguchi, S., & Knight, R.T. (1991). Age effects on the P300 to novel somatosensory stimuli. *Electroencephalography and Clinical Neurophysiology, 78,* 297-301.

Chapter 2

Avolio, B.J., & Waldman, D.A. (1990). An examination of age and cognitive test performance across job complexity and occupational types. *Journal of Applied Psychology, 75,* 43-50.

Avolio, B., & Waldman, D. (1994). Variations in cognitive, perceptual, and psychomotor abilities across the working life span: Examining the effects of race, sex, experience, education, and occupational type. *Psychology and Aging, 9,* 430-442.

Baddeley, A. (1986). *Working memory.* Oxford, England: Clarendon Press.

Ball, K., Berch, D.B., Helmers, K.F., Jobe, J.B., Leveck, M.D., Marsiske, M., et al. (2002). Effects of cognitive training interventions with older adults. A randomized controlled trial. *Journal of the American Medical Association, 288*(18), 2271-2281.

Bosma, H., van Boxtel, M.P.J., Ponds, R.W.H.M., Houx, P., & Jolles, J. (2003). Education and age-related cognitive decline: The contribution of mental workload. *Educational Gerontology, 29,* 165-173.

Bosma, H., van Boxtel, M.P.J., Ponds, R.W.H.M., Jelicic, M., Houx, P., Metesemakers, J., et al. (2002). Engaged lifestyle and cognitive function in middle and old-aged, non-demented persons: A reciprocal association? *Journal for Gerontology and Geriatrics, 35*(6), 575-581.

Crowe, M., Andel, R., Pedersen, N.L., Johansson, B., & Gatz, M. (2003). Does participation in leisure activities lead to reduced risk of Alzheimer's disease? *Journal of Gerontology, 58B*(5), 249-255.

Dartigues, J.F., Gagon, M., Letenneur, L., Barberger-Gateau, P., Commenges, D., Evaldre, M., et al. (1992). Principal lifetime occupation and cognitive impairment in a French elderly cohort. *American Journal of Epidemiology, 135*(9), 981-989.

Friedland, R.P., Fritsch, T., Smyth, K.A., Koss, E., Lerner, A.L., Chen, C.H., et al. (2001). Patients with Alzheimer's disease have reduced activities in midlife compared with healthy control-group members. *Proceedings of the National Academy of Sciences, 98*(6), 3440-3445.

Hambrick, D.Z., Salthouse, T.A., & Meinz, E.J. (1999). Predictors of crossword puzzle proficiency and moderators of age-cognition relations. *Journal of Experimental Psychology: General, 128,* 131-164.

Helmer, C., Letenneur, L., Rouch, I., Richard-Harston, S., Barberger-Gateau, P., Fabrigoule, C., et al. (2001). Occupation during life and risk of dementia in French elderly community residents. *Journal of Neurology, Neurosurgery, and Psychiatry, 71,* 303-309.

Hertzog, C., Hultsch, D.F., & Dixon, R.A. (1999). On the problem of detecting effects of lifestyle on cognitive change in adulthood. *Psychology and Aging, 14,* 528-534.

References

Hultsch, D.F., Hertzog, C., Small, B.J., & Dixon, R.A. (1999). Use it or lose it: Engaged lifestyle as a buffer of cognitive decline in aging? *Psychology and Aging, 14,* 245-263.

Kohn, M.L., & Schooler, C. (1978). The reciprocal effects of the substantive complexity of work and intellectual flexibility: A longitudinal assessment. *American Journal of Sociology, 84,* 24-52.

Kohn, M.L., & Schooler, C. (1983). *Work and personality: An inquiry into the impact of social stratification.* Norwood, NJ: Ablex.

Kohn, M.L., & Slomczyski, K.M. (1990). *Social structure and self-direction: A comparative analysis of the United States and Poland.* Oxford: Basil Blackwell.

Kohn, M.L., Slomczynski, K.M., Janicka, K., Khmelko, V., et al. (1997). Social structure and personality under conditions of radical social change: A comparative analysis of Poland and Ukraine. *American Sociological Review, 62*(4), 614-638.

Kohn, M.L., Zaborowski, W., Janicka, K., Mach, B.W., Khmelko, V., Slomczynski, K.M., et al. (2000). Complexity of activities and personality under conditions of radical social change: A comparative analysis of Poland and Ukraine. *Social Psychology Quarterly, 63*(3), 187-207.

Miller, J., Schooler, C., Kohn, M.L., & Miller, K.A. (1979). Women and work: The psychological effects of occupational conditions. *American Journal of Sociology, 85,* 66-94.

Miller, J., Slomczynski, K.M., & Kohn, M.L. (1985). Continuity of learning-generalization: The effect of job on men's intellective process in the United States and Poland. *American Journal of Sociology, 91,* 593-615.

Miller, K.A., & Kohn, M.L. (1983). The reciprocal effects of job conditions and the intellectuality of leisure-time activities. In M.L. Kohn & C. Schooler (Eds.), *Work and personality: An inquiry into the impact of social stratification* (pp. 217-241). Norwood, NJ: Ablex.

Miller, K.A., Kohn, M.L., & Schooler, C. (1986). Educational self-direction and personality. *American Sociological Review, 51,* 372-390.

Mohammed, A.H., Zhu, S.W., Darmopil, S., Hjerling-Leffler, J., Ernfors, P., Winblad, B., et al. (2002). Environmental enrichment and the brain. *Progress in Brain Research, 138,* 109-133.

Naoi, A., & Schooler, C. (1985). Occupational conditions and psychological functioning in Japan. *American Journal of Sociology, 90,* 729-752.

Naoi, M., & Schooler, C. (1990). Psychological consequences of occupational conditions among Japanese wives. *Social Psychology Quarterly, 58,* 100-116.

Pushkar, D., Etezadi, J., Andres, D., Arbuckle, T., Schwartzman, A.E., & Chaikelson, J. (1999). Models of intelligence in late life: Comment on Hultsch et al. *Psychology and Aging, 14,* 520-527.

Pushkar Gold, D., Cohen, C., Shulman, K., Zucchero, C., Andres, D., & Etezadi, J. (1995). Caregiving and dementia: Predicting negative and positive outcomes for caregivers. *International Journal of Aging & Human Development, 41(3),* 183-201.

References

Qiu, C., Karp, A., von Strauss, E., Winblad, B., Fratiglioni, L., & Bellander, T. (2003). Lifetime principal occupation and risk of Alzheimer's disease in the Kungsholmen Project. *American Journal of Industrial Medicine, 43,* 204-211.

Salthouse, T.A. (1991). Mediation of adult age differences in cognition by reductions in working memory and speed of processing. *Psychological Science, 2,* 179-183.

Salthouse, T.A., Berish, D.E., & Miles, J.D. (2002). The role of cognitive stimulation on the relations between age and cognitive functioning. *Psychology and Aging, 17*(4), 548-557.

Schooler, C. (1984). Psychological effects of complex environments during the life span: A review and theory. *Intelligence, 8,* 259-281.

Schooler, C. (1990). Psychosocial factors and effective cognitive functioning through the life span. In J.E. Birren & K.W. Schaie (Eds.), *Handbook of the psychology of aging* (pp. 347-358). Orlando, FL: Academic Press.

Schooler, C., Miller, J., Miller, K.A., & Richtand, C.N. (1984). Work for the household: Its nature and consequences for husbands and wives. *American Journal of Sociology, 90,* 97-124.

Schooler, C., & Mulatu, M.S. (2001). The reciprocal effects of leisure time activities and intellectual functioning in older people: A longitudinal analysis. *Psychology and Aging, 16,* 466-482.

Schooler, C., Mulatu, M.S., & Oates, G. (1999). The continuing effects of substantively complex work on the intellectual functioning of older workers. *Psychology and Aging, 14*(3), 483-506.

Schooler, C., Mulatu, M.S., & Oates, G. (2004). Effects of occupational self-direction on the intellectual functioning and self-directed orientations of older workers: Findings and implications for individuals and societies. *American Journal of Sociology.*

Schooler, C., & Naoi, M. (1988). The psychological effects of traditional and of economically peripheral job settings in Japan. *American Journal of Sociology, 94*(2), 335-355.

Snowden, D.A., Kemper, S.J., Mortimer, J.T., Greiner, L.H., Wekstein, D.R., & Marksbery, W.R. (1996). Linguistic ability in early life and cognitive function and Alzheimer's disease in late life. *Journal of the American Medical Association, 275,* 528-532.

Spector, A., Thorgrimsen, L., Woods, B., Royan, L., Davies, S., Butterworth, M., et al. (2003). Efficacy of an evidence-based cognitive stimulation therapy programme for people with dementia. *British Journal of Psychiatry, 183,* 248-254.

Stern, Y., Gurland, B., Tatemichi, T.K., Tang, M.X., Wilder, D., & Mayeux, R. (1994). Influence of education and occupation on the incidence of Alzheimer's disease. *Journal of the American Medical Association, 272*(18), 1405-1406.

United States Department of Labor. (1965). *Dictionary of occupational titles* (3rd ed.). Washington, DC: U.S. Government Printing Office.

Verghese, J., Lipton, R.B., Katz, M.J., Hall, C.B., Derby, C.A., Kuslansky, G., et al. (2003). Leisure activities and the risk of dementia in the elderly. *New England Journal of Medicine, 348,* 2508-2516.

Wang, H.-X., Karp, A., Winblad, B., & Fratiglioni, L. (2002). Late-life engagement in social and leisure activities is associated with a decreased risk of dementia: A longitudinal study from the Kungsholmen Project. *American Journal of Epidemiology, 155,* 1081-1087.

Willis, S.L., & Schaie, K.W. (1986). Training the elderly on the ability factors of spatial orientation and inductive reasoning. *Psychology and Aging, 1,* 239-247.

Wilson, R.S., Mendes de Leon, C.F., Barnes, L.L., Schneider, J.A., Bienias, J.L., Evans, D.A., et al. (2002). Participation in cognitively stimulating activities and risk of incident Alzheimer's disease. *Journal of the American Medical Association, 287,* 742-748.

Witkin, H.A., Dyk, R.B., Faterson, H.F., Goodenough, D.R., & Karp, S.A. (1962). *Psychological differentiation: Studies of development.* New York: Wiley.

Chapter 3

Arbuckle, T.Y., Gold, D.P., Andres, D., Schwartzman, A., & Chaikelson, J. (1992). The role of psychosocial context, age, and intelligence in memory performance of older men. *Psychology and Aging, 7,* 25-36.

Ball, K., Berch, D.B., Helmers, K.F., Jobe, J.B., Leveck, M.D., Marsiske, M., et al. (2002). Effects of cognitive training interventions with older adults. A randomized controlled trial. *Journal of the American Medical Association, 288*(18), 2271-2281.

Barnes, L.L., Mendes de Leon, C.F., Wilson, R.S., Bienias, J.L., & Evans, D.A. (2004). Social resources and cognitive decline in a population of older African Americans and Whites. *Neurology, 63,* 2322-2326.

Bassuk, S.S., Glass, T.A., & Berkman, L.F. (1999). Social disengagement and incident cognitive decline in community-dwelling elderly persons. *Annals of Internal Medicine, 131,* 165-173.

Bosma, H., van Boxtel, P.J., Ponds, R.W.H.M., Houx, P.J., Burdorf, A., & Jolles, J. (2003). Mental work demands protect against cognitive impairment: MAAS prospective cohort study. *Experimental Aging Research, 29,* 33-45.

Cabeza, R. (2002). Hemispheric asymmetry reduction in older adults: The HAROLD model. *Psychology and Aging, 17,* 85-100.

Camp, C.J., Bird, M.J., & Cherry, K.E. (2000). Retrieval strategies as a rehabilitation aid for cognitive loss in pathological aging. In R.D. Hill, L. Backman, & A. Stigsdotter Neely (Eds.), *Cognitive Rehabilitation in Old Age* (pp. 224-248). New York: Oxford University Press.

Camp, C.J., Foss, J.W., O'Hanlon, A.M., & Stevens, A.B. (1996). Memory interventions for persons with dementia. *Applied Cognitive Psychology, 10,* 193-210.

Cepeda, N.J., Kramer, A.F., & Gonzalez de Sather, J.C.M. (2001). Changes in executive control across the life span: Examination of task-switching performance. *Developmental Psychology, 37,* 715-730.

Cherry, K.E., & Simmons-D'Gerolamo, S.S. (1999). Effects of a target object orientation task on recall in older adults with probable Alzheimer's disease. *Clinical Gerontologist, 20,* 39-63.

Cherry, K.E., & Simmons-D'Gerolamo, S.S. (2005). Long term effectiveness of spaced-retrieval memory training for older adults with probable Alzheimer's disease. *Experimental Aging Research, 31,* 261-289.

Cherry, K.E., & Smith, A.D. (1998). Normal memory aging. In M. Hersen & V. Van Hasselt (Eds.), *Handbook of Clinical Geropsychology* (pp. 87-110). New York: Plenum Press.

Christensen, H. (1994). Age differences in tests of intelligence and memory in high and low ability subjects: A second sample of eminent academics and scientists. *Personality and Individual Differences, 16,* 919-929.

Christensen, H., Henderson, A.S., Griffiths, K., & Levings, C. (1997). Does ageing inevitably lead to declines in cognitive performance? A longitudinal study of elite academics. *Personality and Individual Differences, 23,* 67-78.

Colcombe, S.J., Erickson, K.I., Raz, N., Webb, A.G., Cohen, N.J., McAuley, E., & Kramer, A.F. (2003). Aerobic fitness reduces brain tissue loss in aging humans. *Journal of Gerontology: Medical Sciences, 58A,* 176-180.

Colcombe, S., & Kramer, A.F. (2003). Fitness effects on the cognitive function of older adults: A meta-analytic study. *Psychological Science, 14,* 125-130.

Craik, F.I.M. (1983). On the transfer of information from temporary to permanent memory. *Philosophical Transactions of the Royal Society of London B, 302,* 341-359.

Crowe, M., Andel, R., Pedersen, N.L., Johansson, B., & Gatz, M. (2003). Does participation in leisure activities lead to reduced risk of Alzheimer's disease? A prospective study of Swedish twins. *Journal of Gerontology: Psychological Sciences, 58B,* 249-255.

Daselaar, S.M., Veltman, D.J., Rombouts, S.A., Raaijmakers, J.G., & Jonker, C. (2003). Deep processing activates the medial temporal lobe in young but not elderly adults. *Neurobiology of Aging, 24,* 1005-1011.

Draganski, B., Gaser, C., Busch, V., Schuierer, G., Bogdahn, U., & May, A., (2004). Neuroplasticity: Changes in grey matter induced by training. *Nature, 427,* 311-312.

Fabrigoule, C., Letenneur, L., Dartigues, J.F., Zarrouk, M., Commenges, D., Barberger-Gateau, P. (1995). Social and leisure activities and risk of dementia: A prospective longitudinal study. *Journal of the American Geriatrics Society, 43,* 485-490.

Fratiglioni, L., Wang, H., Ericsson, K., Maytan, M., & Winblad, B. (2000). Influence of social network on occurrence of dementia: A community-based longitudinal study. *Lancet, 355,* 1315-1319.

References

Gutchess, A.H., Welsh, R.C., Hedden, T., Bangert, A., Minear, M., Liu, L., & Park, D.C. (2005). Aging and the neural correlates of successful picture encoding: Frontal activations compensate for decreased medial-temporal activity. *Journal of Cognitive Neuroscience, 17(1),* 84-96.

Hambrick, D.Z., Salthouse, T.A., & Meinz, E.J. (1999). Predictors of crossword puzzle proficiency and moderators of age-cognition relations. *Journal of Experimental Psychology: General, 128,* 131-164.

Hasher, L., & Zacks, R. (1979). Automatic and effortful processes in memory. *Journal of Experimental Psychology: General, 108,* 356-388.

Hedden, T., Lautenschlager, G.J., & Park, D.C. (2005). Contributions of processing ability and knowledge to verbal memory tasks across the adult lifespan. *Quarterly Journal of Experimental Psychology, 58A,* 169-190.

Hultsch, D.F., Hertzog, C., Small, B.J., & Dixon, R.A. (1999). Use it or lose it: Engaged lifestyle as a buffer of cognitive decline in aging? *Psychology and Aging, 14,* 245-263.

Kramer, A.F., Hahn, S., Cohen, N.J., Banich, M.T., McAuley, E., Harrison, C.R., Chason, J., Vakil, E., Bardell, L., Boileau, R.A., & Colcombe, A. (1999). Ageing, fitness and neurocognitive function. *Nature, 400,* 418-419.

Liu, L.L., & Park, D.C. (2004). Aging and medial adherence: The use of automatic processes to achieve effortful things. *Psychology and Aging, 19,* 318-325.

Marsiske, M. (2005). Cognitive interventions with older adults: The transfer challenge. Talk presented at the International Conference on the Future of Cognitive Aging Research, University Park, PA.

Nyberg, L., Sandblom, J., Jones, S., Neely, A.S., Petersson, K.M., Ingvar, M., & Backman, L. (2003). Neural correlates of training-related memory improvement in adulthood and aging. *Proceedings of the National Academy of Sciences, 100,* 13728-13733.

Park, D.C. (2000). The basic mechanism accounting for age-related decline in cognitive function. In D.C. Park & N. Schwarz (Eds.), *Cognitive Aging: A Primer.* Philadelphia: Psychology Press.

Park, D.C., Lautenschlager, G., Hedden, T., Davidson, N., Smith, A.D., & Smith, P. (2002). Models of visuospatial and verbal memory across the adult life span. *Psychology and Aging, 17(2),* 299-320.

Park, D.C., Polk, T.A., Mikels, J.A., Taylor, S.F., & Marchuetz, C. (2001). Cerebral aging: Brain and behavior models of cognitive function. *Dialogues in Clinical Neuroscience, 3,* 151-165.

Park, D.C., Smith, A.D., Lautenschlager, G., Earles, J., Frieske, D., Zwahr, M., & Gaines, C. (1996). Mediators of long-term memory performance across the life span. *Psychology and Aging, 11,* 621-637.

Park, D.C., Welsh, R.C., Marshuetz, C., Gutchess, A.H., Mikels, J., Polk, T.A., Noll, D.C., & Taylor, S.F. (2003). Working memory for complex scenes: Age differences in frontal and hippocampal activations. *Journal of Cognitive Neuroscience, 15,* 1122-1134.

Pushkar Gold, D., Andres, D., Etezadi, J., Arbuckle, T., Schwartzman, A., & Chaikelson, J. (1995). Structural equation modeling of intellectual change and continuity and predictors of intelligence in older men. *Psychology and Aging, 10,* 294-303.

Raz, N. (2000). Aging of the brain and its impact on cognitive performance: Integration of structural and functional findings. In F.I. Craik & T.A. Salthouse (Eds.), *Handbook of Aging and Cognition* (2nd ed., pp. 1-90). Mahwah, NJ: Erlbaum.

Resnick, S.M., Goldszal, A.F., Davatzikos, C., Golski, S., Kraut, M.A., Metter, E.J., Bryan, R.N., & Zonderman, A.B. (2000). One-year age changes in MRI brain volumes in older adults. *Cerebral Cortex, 10,* 464-472.

Resnick, S.M., Pham, D.L., Kraut, M.A., Zonderman, A.B., & Davatzikos, C. (2003). Longitudinal magnetic resonance imaging studies of older adults: A shrinking brain. *Journal of Neuroscience, 8,* 3295-3301.

Reuter-Lorenz, P.A. (2002). New visions of the aging mind and brain. *Trends in Cognitive Sciences, 6,* 394-400.

Roenker, D.L., Cissell, G.M., Ball, K.K., Wadley, V.G., & Edwards, J.D. (2003). Speed-of-processing and driving simulator training result in improved driving performance. *Human Factors, 45,* 218-233.

Rosen, A.C., Prull, M.W., O'Hara, R., Race, E.A., Desmond, J.E., Glover, G.H., Yesavage, J.A., & Gabrieli, J.D.E. (2002). Variable effects of aging on frontal lobe contributions to memory. *Neuroreport, 13,* 2425-2428.

Salthouse, T.A. (1996). The processing-speed theory of adult age differences in cognition. *Psychological Review, 103,* 403-428.

Salthouse, T.A. (in press). Mental exercise and aging: Evaluating the validity of the "Use it or lose it" hypothesis. *Perspectives in Psychological Science.*

Salthouse, T.A., Babcock, R., Skovronek, E., Mitchell, D., & Palmon, R. (1990). Age and experience effects in spatial visualization. *Developmental Psychology, 26,* 128-136.

Salthouse, T.A., Berish, D.E., & Miles, J.D. (2002). The role of cognitive stimulation on the relations between age and cognitive functioning. *Psychology and Aging, 17,* 548-557.

Salthouse, T.A., & Mitchell, D.R.D. (1990). Effects of age and naturally occurring experience on spatial visualization performance. *Developmental Psychology, 26,* 845-854.

Scarmea, N., Levy, G., Tang, M.-X., Manly, J., & Stern, Y. (2001). Influence of leisure activity on the incidence of Alzheimer's disease. *Neurology, 57,* 2236-2242.

Schooler, C., Mulatu, M.S., & Oates, G. (1999). The continuing effects of substantively complex work on the intellectual functioning of older workers. *Psychology and Aging, 14,* 483-506.

Seidler, A., Bernhardt, T., Nienhaus, A., & Frolich, L. (2003). Association between the psychosocial network and dementia—a case-control study. *Journal of Psychiatric Research, 37,* 89-98.

Shimamura, A.P., Berry, J.M., Mangels, J.A., Rustings, C.L., & Jurica, P.J. (1995). Memory and cognitive abilities in university professors: Evidence for successful aging. *Psychological Science, 6,* 271-277.

Wang, H., Karp, A., Winblad, B., & Fratiglioni, L. (2002). Late-life engagement in leisure activities is associated with a decreased risk of dementia: A longitudinal study from the Kungsholmen project. *American Journal of Epidemiology, 155,* 1081-1087.

Willis, S.L., Jay, G.M., Diehl, M., & Marsiske, M. (1992). Longitudinal change and prediction of everyday task competence in the elderly. *Research on Aging, 14,* 68-91.

Willis, S.L., & Schaie, K.W. (1986). Training the elderly on the ability factors of spatial orientation and inductive reasoning. *Psychology and Aging, 1,* 239-247.

Wilson, R.S., Barnes, L.L., & Bennett, D.A. (2003). Assessment of lifetime participation in cognitively stimulating activities. *Journal of Clinical and Experimental Neuropsychology, 25,* 634-642.

Wilson, R.S., Bennett, D.A., Beckett, L.A., Morris, M.C., Gilley, D.W., Bienias, J.L., Scherr, P.A., & Evans, D.A. (1999). Cognitive activity in older persons from a geographically defined population. *Journal of Gerontology: Series B: Psychological Sciences and Social Sciences, 54B,* P155-P160.

Wilson, R.S., Bennett, D.A. Bienias, J.L., Aggarwal, N.T., Mendes De Leon, C.F., Morris, M.C., et al. (2002). Cognitive activity and incident AD in a population-based sample of older persons. *Neurology, 59*(12), 1910-1914.

Wilson, R.S., Mendes De Leon, C.F., Barnes, L.L., Scneider, J.A., Bienias, J.L., Evans, D.A., et al. (2002). Participation in cognitively stimulating activities and risk of incident Alzheimer's disease. *Journal of the American Medical Association, 287,* 742-748.

Chapter 4

Ackerman, P.L. (1994). Intelligence, attention, and learning: Maximal and typical performance. In D.K. Detterman (Ed.), *Current topics in human intelligence:* Vol. 4. *Theories of intelligence* (pp. 1-27). Norwood, NJ: Ablex.

Ackerman, P.L., & Rolfhus, E.L. (1999). The locus of adult intelligence: Knowledge, abilities, and nonability traits. *Psychology and Aging, 14,* 314-330.

Adams, M.J., Tenney, Y.J., & Pew, R.W. (1995). Situation awareness and the cognitive management of complex systems. *Human Factors, 37,* 85-104.

Anderson, J.R. (1990). *The adaptive character of thought.* Hillsdale, NJ: Erlbaum.

References

Ball, K., Berch, D.B., Helmers, K.F., Jobe, J.B., Leveck, M.D., Marsiske, M., Morris, J.N., Rebok, G.W., Smith, D.M., Tennstedt, S.L., Unverzagt, F.W., & Willis, S.L. (2002). Effects of cognitive training interventions with older adults: A randomized controlled trial. *Journal of the American Medical Association, 288,* 2271-2281.

Baltes, P.B., & Staudinger, U.M. (1993). The search for a psychology of wisdom. *Current Directions in Psychological Science, 2,* 75-80.

Bellenkes, M.A., Wickens, C.D., & Kramer, A.F. (1997). Visual scanning and pilot expertise: The role of attentional flexibility and mental model development. *Aviation, Space, and Environmental Medicine, 68,* 569-579.

Bjork, R.A. (1999). Assessing our own competence: Heuristics and illusions. In D. Gopher and A. Koriat (Eds.), *Attention and performance XVII. Cognitive regulation of performance: Interaction of theory and application* (pp. 435-459). Cambridge, MA: MIT Press.

Bosman, E.A. (1993). Age-related differences in motoric aspects of transcription typing skill. *Psychology and Aging, 8,* 87-102.

Bosman, E.A., & Charness, N. (1996). Age-related differences in skilled performance and skill acquisition. In F. Blanchard-Fields & T.M. Hess (Eds.), *Perspectives on cognitive change in adulthood and aging* (pp. 428-453). New York: McGraw-Hill.

Broach, D., & Schroeder, D.J. (2006). Air traffic control specialist age and en route operational errors. *International Journal of Aviation Psychology, 16,* 363-374.

Charness, N. (1981). Visual short-term memory and aging in chess players. *Journal of Gerontology, 36,* 615-619.

Charness, N., Reingold, E.M., Pomplun, M., & Stampe, D.M. (2001). The perceptual aspect of skilled performance in chess: Evidence from eye movements. *Memory and Cognition, 29,* 1146-1152.

Clancy, S.M., & Hoyer, W.J. (1994). Age and skill in visual search. *Developmental Psychology, 30,* 545-552.

Colcombe, S.J., Kramer, A.F., Erickson, K.I., Scalf, P., McAuley, E., Cohen, N.J., Webb, A., Jerome, G.J., Marquez, D.X., & Elavsky, S. (2004). Cardiovascular fitness, cortical plasticity, and aging. *Proceedings of the National Academy of Sciences USA, 101*(9), 3316-3321.

Colonia-Willner, R. (1998). Practical intelligence at work: Relationship between aging and cognitive efficiency among managers in a bank environment. *Psychology and Aging, 13,* 45-57.

Craik, F.I.M., & Jennings, J.M. (1992). Human memory. In F.I.M. Craik & T.A. Salthouse (Eds.), *The handbook of aging and cognition* (pp. 51-110). Hillsdale, NJ: Erlbaum.

Diehl, M. (1998). Everyday competence in later life: Current status and future directions. *Gerontologist, 38,* 422-433.

Ericsson, K.A., & Kintsch, W. (1995). Long-term working memory. *Psychological Review, 102,* 211-245.

References

Ericsson, K.A., & Lehmann, A.C. (1996). Expert and exceptional performance: Evidence of maximal adaptation to task constraints. *Annual Review of Psychology, 47,* 273-305.

Ericsson, K.A., Patel, V.L., & Kintsch, W. (2000). How experts' adaptations to representative task demands account for the expertise effect in memory recall: Comment on Vicente and Wang (1998). *Psychological Review, 107,* 587-592.

Feigenbaum, E.A. (1989). What hath Simon wrought? In D. Klahr & K. Kotovsky (Eds.), *Complex information processing: The impact of Herbert A. Simon* (pp. 165-180). Hillsdale, NJ: Erlbaum.

Glaser, R., & Chi, M. (1988). Overview. In M. Chi, R. Glaser, & M.J. Farr (Eds.), *The nature of expertise* (pp. xv-xxvii). Hillsdale, NJ: Hove & London.

Halpern, A.R., Bartlett, J.C., & Dowling, W.J. (1995). Aging and experience in the recognition of musical transpositions. *Psychology and Aging, 10,* 325-342.

Hambrick, D.Z., & Engle, R.W. (2002). Effects of domain knowledge, working memory capacity, and age on cognitive performance: An investigation of the knowledge-is-power hypothesis. *Cognitive Psychology, 44,* 339-387.

Hardy, D., & Parasuraman, R. (1997). Cognition and flight performance in older pilots. *Journal of Experimental Psychology: Applied, 3,* 313-348.

Hershey, D.A., Jacobs-Lawson, J.M., & Walsh, D.A. (2003). Influences of age and training on script development. *Aging, Neuropsychology, and Cognition, 10,* 1-19.

Hess, T.M., Osowski, N.L., & Leclerc, C.M. (2005). Age and experience influences on the complexity of social inferences. *Psychology and Aging, 20,* 447-449.

Hoffman, R.R., Shadbolt, N.R., Burton, A.M., & Klein, G. (1995). Eliciting knowledge from experts: A methodological analysis. *Organizational Behavior and Human Decision Processes, 62,* 129-158.

Hoyer, W.J., & Ingolfsdottir, D. (2003). Age, skill, and contextual cuing in target detection. *Psychology and Aging, 18,* 210-218.

Hutchins, E. (1995). How a cockpit remembers its speed. *Cognitive Science, 19,* 265-288.

Jastrzembski, T., Charness, N., & Vasyukova, C. (2006). Expertise and age effects on knowledge activation in chess. *Psychology and Aging, 21,* 401-405.

Jenkins, J. (1979). Four points to remember: A tetrahedral model and memory experiments. In L.S. Cermak & F.I.M. Craik (Eds.), *Levels of processing in human memory.* Mahwah, NJ: Erlbaum.

Kirlik, A. (1995). Requirements for psychological models to support design: Towards ecological task analysis. In J.M. Flach, P.A. Hancock, J.K. Caird, & K.J. Vicente (Eds.), *An ecological approach to human-machine systems I: A global perspective* (pp. 68-120). Hillsdale, NJ: Erlbaum.

Korniotis, G., & Kumar, A. (2005). Does investment skill decline due to cognitive aging or improve with experience? Unpublished paper.

References

Kramer, A.F., Larish, J., Weber, T., & Bardell, L. (1999). Training for executive control: Task coordination strategies and aging. In D. Gopher & A. Koriat (Eds.), *Attention and performance XVII*. Cambridge, MA: MIT Press.

Krampe, R.T., Engbert, R., & Kliegl, R. (2002). The effects of expertise and age on rhythm production: Adaptations to timing and sequencing constraints. *Brain and Cognition, 48*, 179-194.

Krampe, R., & Ericsson, K.A. (1996). Maintaining excellence: Deliberate practice and elite performance in younger and older pianists. *Journal of Experimental Psychology: General, 125*, 331-359.

Lassiter, D., Morrow, D.G., Hinson, G., Miller, M., & Hambrick, D. (1997). Expertise and age effects on pilot mental workload in a simulated aviation task. In W.A. Rogers (Ed.), *Designing for an aging population: Ten years of human factors/ergonomics research* (pp. 226-230). Santa Monica, CA: Human Factors and Ergonomics Society.

Lawton, M.P. (1982). Competence, environmental press, and the adaptation of older people. In M.P. Lawton, P.G. Windley, & T.O. Byerts (Eds.), *Aging and the environment: Theoretical approaches* (pp. 33-59). New York: Springer.

Li, G., Baker, S.P., Grabowski, J.G., Rebok, G.W., et al. (2003). Age, flight experience, and risk of crash involvement in a cohort of professional pilots. *American Journal of Epidemiology, 157*, 874-880.

Li, G., Grabowski, J.G., Baker, S.P., & Rebok, G.W. (2006). Pilot error in air carrier accidents: Does age matter? *Aviation, Space, and Environmental Medicine, 77*, 737-741.

Lindenberger, U., Kliegl, R., & Baltes, P.B. (1992). Professional expertise does not eliminate age differences in imagery-based memory performance during adulthood. *Psychology and Aging, 7*, 585-593.

Lobjois, R., Benguigui, N., & Bertsch, J. (2005). Aging and tennis playing in a coincidence-timing task with an accelerating object: The role of visuomotor delay. *Research Quarterly for Exercise and Sport, 76*, 398-406.

Masunaga, H., & Horn, J. (2001). Expertise and age-related changes in components of intelligence. *Psychology and Aging, 16*, 293-311.

Meinz, E.J. (2000). Experience-based attenuation of age-related differences in music cognition tasks. *Psychology and Aging, 15*, 297-312.

Meinz, E.J., & Salthouse, T.A. (1998). The effects of age and experience on memory for visually presented music. *Journal of Gerontology: Psychological Sciences, 53*, 60-69.

Miller, L.M.S., Stine-Morrow, E.A.L., Kirkorian, H., & Conroy, M. (2004). Age differences in knowledge-driven reading. *Journal of Educational Psychology, 96*, 811-821.

Morrow, D.G., Leirer, V.O., & Altieri, P.A. (1992). Aging, expertise, and narrative processing. *Psychology and Aging, 7*, 376-388.

Morrow, D.G., Leirer, V., Altiere, P., & Fitzsimmons, C. (1994). When expertise reduces age differences in performance. *Psychology and Aging, 9,* 134-148.

Morrow, D.G., Miller, L., Ridolfo, H.E., Kokayeff, N., Chang, D., Fischer, U., & Stine-Morrow, E.A.L. (2004). Expertise and age differences in a pilot decision making task. *Proceedings of the Human Factors and Ergonomics Society 48th annual meeting.* Santa Monica, CA: Human Factors and Ergonomics Society.

Morrow, D.G., Miller, L.S., Ridolfo, H.E., Menard, W., Stine-Morrow, E.A.L., & Magnor, C. (2005). Environmental support for older and younger pilots' comprehension of Air Traffic Control information. *Journal of Gerontology: Psychological Sciences, 60B,* P11-P18.

Morrow, D.G., Ridolfo, H.E., Menard, W.E., Sanborn, A., Stine-Morrow, E.A.L., Magnor, C., Herman, L., Teller, T., & Bryant, D. (2003). Environmental support promotes expertise-based mitigation of age differences in pilot communication tasks. *Psychology and Aging, 18,* 268-284.

Morrow, D.G., Wickens, C.D., Rantanen, E.M., Chang, D., & Marcus, J. (2008). Designing external aids that support older pilots' communication. *International Journal of Aviation Psychology, 18,* 167-182.

Murrell, F.H. (1970). The effect of extensive practice on age differences in reaction time. *Journal of Gerontology, 25,* 268-274.

Nunes, A. (2006). Assessing the degree to which domain specific experience can offset age-related decline on basic cognitive abilities and complex task performance. PhD dissertation, University of Illinois at Urbana-Champaign.

Orasanu, J., & Fischer, U. (1997). Finding decisions in natural environments: The view from the cockpit. In C. Zsambok & G.A. Klein (Eds.), *Naturalistic decision-making* (pp. 343-357). Mahwah, NJ: Erlbaum.

Park, D.C. (1994). Aging, cognition, and work. *Human Performance, 7,* 181-205.

Park, D.C., Smith, A.D., Lautenschlager, G., Earles, J.L., Frieske, D., Zwahr, M., & Gaines, C.L. (1996). Mediators of long-term memory performance across the life span. *Psychology and Aging, 11,* 621-637.

Rybash, J.M., Hoyer, W.J., & Roodin, P.A. (1986). *Adult cognition and aging: Developmental changes in processing, knowing and thinking.* New York: Pergamon Press.

Salthouse, T.A. (1984). Effects of age and skill in typing. *Journal of Experimental Psychology, 113,* 345-371.

Salthouse, T.A. (1990). Influence of experience on age difference in cognitive functioning. *Human Factors, 32,* 551-569.

Salthouse, T.A. (1991). *Theoretical perspectives on cognitive aging.* Hillsdale, NJ: Erlbaum.

Salthouse, T.A. (1995). Refining the concept of psychological compensation. In R.A. Dixon & L. Backman (Eds.), *Compensating for psychological deficits and declines: Managing losses and promoting gains* (21-34). Mahwah, NJ: Erlbaum.

Salthouse, T.A., Babcock, R., Skovronek, E., Mitchell, D., & Palmon, R. (1990). Age and experience effects in spatial visualization. *Developmental Psychology, 26,* 128-136.

Salthouse, T.A., & Maurer, J.J. (1996). Aging, job performance, and career development. In J.E. Birren & K.W. Schaie (Eds.), *Handbook of the psychology of aging* (4th ed., pp. 353-364). New York: Academic Press.

Schooler, C., Mulatu, M.S., & Oates, C. (1999). Reciprocal effects of substantive complexity of work and cognitive function among older workers. *Psychology and Aging, 14,* 483-506.

Schultz, R., & Curnow, C. (1988). Peak performance and age among superatheletes: Track and field, swimming, baseball, tennis, and golf. *Journal of Gerontology: Psychological Sciences, 43,* P113-P120.

Shanteau, J. (1992). How much information does an expert use? Is it relevant? *Acta Psychologica, 81,* 75-86.

Sirven, J.I., & Morrow, D.G. (2007). Fly the graying skies: A question of competency vs. age (editorial). *Neurology, 68,* 630-631.

Stern, P., & Carstensen, L. (2000). *The aging mind: Opportunities in cognitive research.* Washington, DC: National Academy Press.

Stine-Morrow, E.A.L., Parisi, J., Morrow, D.G., Greene, J., & Park, D.C. (2007). An engagement model of cognitive optimization through adulthood. *Journal of Gerontology: Psychological Sciences, 62B,* 62-69.

Taylor, J.L., Kennedy, Q., Noda, A., & Yesavage, J.A. (2007). Pilot age and expertise predict flight simulator performance: A three-year longitudinal study. *Neurology, 68,* 648-654.

Taylor, J.L., O'Hara, R., Mumenthaler, M.S., Rosen, A.C., & Yesavage, J.A. (2005). Cognitive ability, expertise, and age differences in following Air-Traffic Control instructions. *Psychology and Aging, 20,* 117-132.

Taylor, J., Yesavage, J., Morrow, D.G., Dolhert, N., & Poon, L. (1994). The effects of information load and speech rate on young and older aircraft pilots' ability to execute simulated Air Traffic Controller instructions. *Journal of Gerontology: Psychological Sciences, 49,* P191-P200.

Tsang, P.S. (2003). Assessing cognitive aging in piloting. In P.S. Tsang & M.A. Vidulich (Eds.), *Principles and practice of aviation psychology* (pp. 507-546). Mahwah, NJ: Erlbaum.

Tsang, P.S., & Shaner, T.L. (1998). Age, attention, expertise, and time sharing performance. *Psychology and Aging, 13,* 323-347.

Vicente, K.J., & Wang, J.H. (1998). An ecological theory of expertise effects in memory recall. *Psychological Review, 105,* 33-57.

Chapter 5

Adlard PA, Cotman CW (2004) Voluntary exercise protects against stress-induced decreases in brain-derived neurotrophic factor protein expression. *Neuroscience* 124:985-992.

Adlard PA, Perreau VM, Engesser-Cesar C, Cotman CW (2004) The timecourse of induction of brain-derived neurotrophic factor mRNA and protein in the rat hippocampus following voluntary exercise. *Neurosci Lett* 363:43-48.

Alonso M, Vianna MR, Depino AM, Mello e Souza T, Pereira P, Szapiro G, Viola H, Pitossi F, Izquierdo I, Medina JH (2002a) BDNF-triggered events in the rat hippocampus are required for both short- and long-term memory formation. *Hippocampus* 12:551-560.

Alonso M, Vianna MR, Izquierdo I, Medina JH (2002b) Signaling mechanisms mediating BDNF modulation of memory formation in vivo in the hippocampus. *Cell Mol Neurobiol* 22:663-674.

Anderson BJ, Eckburg PB, Relucio KI (2002) Alterations in the thickness of motor cortical subregions after motor-skill learning and exercise. *Learn Mem* 9:1-9.

Anderson BJ, Gatley SJ, Rapp DN, Coburn-Litvak PS, Volkow ND (2000a) The ratio of striatal D1 to muscarinic receptors changes in aging rats housed in an enriched environment. *Brain Res* 872:262-265.

Anderson BJ, Rapp DN, Baek DH, McCloskey DP, Coburn-Litvak PS, Robinson JK (2000b) Exercise influences spatial learning in the radial arm maze. *Physiol Behav* 70:425-429.

Arida RM, de Jesus Vieira A, Cavalheiro EA (1998) Effect of physical exercise on kindling development. *Epilepsy Res* 30:127-132.

Arida RM, Scorza FA, dos Santos NF, Peres CA, Cavalheiro EA (1999) Effect of physical exercise on seizure occurrence in a model of temporal lobe epilepsy in rats. *Epilepsy Res* 37:45-52.

Babyak M, Blumenthal JA, Herman S, Khatri P, Doraiswamy M, Moore K, Craighead WE, Baldewicz TT, Krishnan KR (2000) Exercise treatment for major depression: maintenance of therapeutic benefit at 10 months. *Psychosom Med* 62:633-638.

Banasr M, Hery M, Printemps R, Daszuta A (2004) Serotonin-induced increases in adult cell proliferation and neurogenesis are mediated through different and common 5-HT receptor subtypes in the dentate gyrus and the subventricular zone. *Neuropsychopharmacology* 29:450-460.

Barnes CA, Forster MJ, Fleshner M, Ahanotu EN, Laudenslager ML, Mazzeo RS, Maier SF, Lal H (1991) Exercise does not modify spatial memory, brain autoimmunity, or antibody response in aged F-344 rats. *Neurobiol Aging* 12:47-53.

Baruch DE, Swain RA, Helmstetter FJ (2004) Effects of exercise on Pavlovian fear conditioning. *Behav Neurosci* 118:1123-1127.

References

Black JE, Isaacs KR, Anderson BJ, Alcantara AA, Greenough WT (1990) Learning causes synaptogenesis, whereas motor activity causes angiogenesis, in cerebellar cortex of adult rats. *Proc Natl Acad Sci* USA 87:5568-5572.

Bland BH, Vanderwolf CH (1972) Electrical stimulation of the hippocampal formation: behavioral and bioelectrical effects. *Brain Res* 43:89-106.

Blumenthal JA, Babyak MA, Moore KA, Craighead WE, Herman S, Khatri P, Waugh R, Napolitano MA, Forman LM, Appelbaum M, Doraiswamy PM, Krishnan KR (1999) Effects of exercise training on older patients with major depression. *Arch Intern Med* 159:2349-2356.

Campisi J, Leem TH, Greenwood BN, Hansen MK, Moraska A, Higgins K, Smith TP, Fleshner M (2003) Habitual physical activity facilitates stress-induced HSP72 induction in brain, peripheral, and immune tissues. *Am J Physiol Regul Integr Comp Physiol* 284:R520-530.

Carro E, Trejo JL, Busiguina S, Torres-Aleman I (2001) Circulating insulin-like growth factor I mediates the protective effects of physical exercise against brain insults of different etiology and anatomy. *J Neurosci* 21:5678-5684.

Chennaoui M, Drogou C, Gomez-Merino D, Grimaldi B, Fillion G, Guezennec CY (2001) Endurance training effects on 5-HT(1B) receptors mRNA expression in cerebellum, striatum, frontal cortex and hippocampus of rats. *Neurosci Lett* 307:33-36.

Colcombe SJ, Erickson KI, Raz N, Webb AG, Cohen NJ, McAuley E, Kramer AF (2003) Aerobic fitness reduces brain tissue loss in aging humans. *J Gerontol A Biol Sci Med Sci* 58:176-180.

Comery TA, Shah R, Greenough WT (1995) Differential rearing alters spine density on medium-sized spiny neurons in the rat corpus striatum: evidence for association of morphological plasticity with early response gene expression. *Neurobiol Learn Mem* 63:217-219.

Czeh B, Michaelis T, Watanabe T, Frahm J, de Biurrun G, van Kampen M, Bartolomucci A, Fuchs E (2001) Stress-induced changes in cerebral metabolites, hippocampal volume, and cell proliferation are prevented by antidepressant treatment with tianeptine. *Proc Natl Acad Sci USA* 98:12796-12801.

Czurko A, Hirase H, Csicsvari J, Buzsaki G (1999) Sustained activation of hippocampal pyramidal cells by "space clamping" in a running wheel. *Eur J Neurosci* 11:344-352.

De Bruin LA, Schasfoort EM, Steffens AB, Korf J (1990) Effects of stress and exercise on rat hippocampus and striatum extracellular lactate. *Am J Physiol* 259:R773-779.

Dimeo F, Bauer M, Varahram I, Proest G, Halter U (2001) Benefits from aerobic exercise in patients with major depression: a pilot study. *Br J Sports Med* 35:114-117.

Ding YH, Young CN, Luan X, Li J, Rafols JA, Clark JC, McAllister JP, 2nd, Ding Y (2005) Exercise preconditioning ameliorates inflammatory injury in ischemic rats during reperfusion. *Acta Neuropathol (Berl)* 109:237-246.

Dishman RK, Dunn AL, Youngstedt SD, Davis JM, Burgess ML, Wilson SP, Wilson MA (1996) Increased open field locomotion and decreased striatal GABA$_A$ binding after activity wheel running. *Physiol Behav* 60:699-705.

Dudar JD, Whishaw IQ, Szerb JC (1979) Release of acetylcholine from the hippocampus of freely moving rats during sensory stimulation and running. *Neuropharmacology* 18:673-678.

Duman RS (2004) Depression: a case of neuronal life and death? *Biol Psychiatry* 56:140-145.

Feng R, Rampon C, Tang YP, Shrom D, Jin J, Kyin M, Sopher B, Miller MW, Ware CB, Martin GM, Kim SH, Langdon RB, Sisodia SS, Tsien JZ (2001) Deficient neurogenesis in forebrain-specific presenilin-1 knockout mice is associated with reduced clearance of hippocampal memory traces. *Neuron* 32:911-926.

Fischer W, Wictorin K, Bjorklund A, Williams LR, Varon S, Gage FH (1987) Amelioration of cholinergic neuron atrophy and spatial memory impairment in aged rats by nerve growth factor. *Nature* 329:65-68.

Fleshner M, Campisi J, Johnson JD (2003) Can exercise stress facilitate innate immunity? A functional role for stress-induced extracellular Hsp72. *Exerc Immunol Rev* 9:6-24.

Fordyce DE, Farrar RP (1991a) Effect of physical activity on hippocampal high affinity choline uptake and muscarinic binding: a comparison between young and old F344 rats. *Brain Res* 541:57-62.

Fordyce DE, Farrar RP (1991b) Physical activity effects on hippocampal and parietal cortical cholinergic function and spatial learning in F344 rats. *Behav Brain Res* 43:115-123.

Fordyce DE, Starnes JW, Farrar RP (1991) Compensation of the age-related decline in hippocampal muscarinic receptor density through daily exercise or underfeeding. *J Gerontol* 46:B245-248.

Fordyce DE, Wehner JM (1993) Physical activity enhances spatial learning performance with an associated alteration in hippocampal protein kinase C activity in C57BL/6 and DBA/2 mice. *Brain Res* 619:111-119.

Gilliam PE, Spirduso WW, Martin TP, Walters TJ, Wilcox RE, Farrar RP (1984) The effects of exercise training on [3H]-spiperone binding in rat striatum. *Pharmacol Biochem Behav* 20:863-867.

Goodwin RD (2003) Association between physical activity and mental disorders among adults in the United States. *Prev Med* 36:698-703.

Greenough WT (1984) Structural correlates of information storage in the mammalian brain: A review and hypothesis. *Trends Neurosci* 7:229-233.

Griesbach GS, Hovda DA, Molteni R, Wu A, Gomez-Pinilla F (2004) Voluntary exercise following traumatic brain injury: brain-derived neurotrophic factor upregulation and recovery of function. *Neuroscience* 125:129-139.

Gross PM, Marcus ML, Heistad DD (1980) Regional distribution of cerebral blood flow during exercise in dogs. *J Appl Physiol* 48:213-217.

References

Isaacs KR, Anderson BJ, Alcantara AA, Black JE, Greenough WT (1992) Exercise and the brain: angiogenesis in the adult rat cerebellum after vigorous physical activity and motor skill learning. *J Cereb Blood Flow Metab* 12:110-119.

Jakubowska-Dogru E, Gumusbas U (2005) Chronic intracerebroventricular NGF administration improves working memory in young adult memory deficient rats. *Neurosci Lett* 382:45-50.

Kanda K, Hashizume K (1998) Effects of long-term physical exercise on age-related changes of spinal motoneurons and peripheral nerves in rats. *Neurosci Res* 31:69-75.

Keller A, Arissian K, Asanuma H (1992) Synaptic proliferation in the motor cortex of adult cats after long-term thalamic stimulation. *J Neurophysiol* 68:295-308.

Kempermann G, Kuhn HG, Gage FH (1997) More hippocampal neurons in adult mice living in an enriched environment. *Nature* 386:493-495.

Kjaer M (1998) Adrenal medulla and exercise training. *Eur J Appl Physiol Occup Physiol* 77:195-199.

Kleim JA, Cooper NR, VandenBerg PM (2002) Exercise induces angiogenesis but does not alter movement representations within rat motor cortex. *Brain Res* 934:1-6.

Kleim JA, Hogg TM, VandenBerg PM, Cooper NR, Bruneau R, Remple M (2004) Cortical synaptogenesis and motor map reorganization occur during late, but not early, phase of motor skill learning. *J Neurosci* 24:628-633.

Kleim JA, Lussnig E, Schwarz ER, Comery TA, Greenough WT (1996) Synaptogenesis and Fos expression in the motor cortex of the adult rat after motor skill learning. *J Neurosci* 16:4529-4535.

Lambert TJ, Fernandez SM, Frick KM (2005) Different types of environmental enrichment have discrepant effects on spatial memory and synaptophysin levels in female mice. *Neurobiol Learn Mem* 83:206-216.

Larsen JO, Skalicky M, Viidik A (2000) Does long-term physical exercise counteract age-related Purkinje cell loss? A stereological study of rat cerebellum. *J Comp Neurol* 428:213-222.

Lee HH, Kim H, Lee MH, Chang HK, Lee TH, Jang MH, Shin MC, Lim BV, Shin MS, Kim YP, Yoon JH, Jeong IG, Kim CJ (2003) Treadmill exercise decreases intrastriatal hemorrhage-induced neuronal cell death via suppression on caspase-3 expression in rats. *Neurosci Lett* 352:33-36.

Li J, Luan X, Clark JC, Rafols JA, Ding Y (2004) Neuroprotection against transient cerebral ischemia by exercise pre-conditioning in rats. *Neurol Res* 26:404-408.

Liddell HS (1925) The relation between maze learning and spontaneous activity in the sheep. J Comp Psychol 5:475-483.

MacRae PG, Spirduso WW, Cartee GD, Farrar RP, Wilcox RE (1987a) Endurance training effects on striatal D2 dopamine receptor binding and striatal dopamine metabolite levels. *Neurosci Lett* 79:138-144.

References

MacRae PG, Spirduso WW, Walters TJ, Farrar RP, Wilcox RE (1987b) Endurance training effects on striatal D2 dopamine receptor binding and striatal dopamine metabolites in presenescent older rats. *Psychopharmacology* 92:236-240.

Malberg JE, Duman RS (2003) Cell proliferation in adult hippocampus is decreased by inescapable stress: reversal by fluoxetine treatment. *Neuropsychopharmacology* 28:1562-1571.

Markowska AL, Price D, Koliatsos VE (1996) Selective effects of nerve growth factor on spatial recent memory as assessed by a delayed nonmatching-to-position task in the water maze. *J Neurosci* 16:3541-3548.

Marsh SA, Coombes JS (2005) Exercise and the endothelial cell. *Int J Cardiol* 99:165-169.

Martinsen EW, Medhus A, Sandvik L (1985) Effects of aerobic exercise on depression: a controlled study. *Br Med J (Clin Res Ed)* 291:109.

McCloskey DP, Adamo DS, Anderson BJ (2001) Exercise increases metabolic capacity in the motor cortex and striatum, but not in the hippocampus. *Brain Res* 891:168-175.

Mizuno M, Yamada K, Olariu A, Nawa H, Nabeshima T (2000) Involvement of brain-derived neurotrophic factor in spatial memory formation and maintenance in a radial arm maze test in rats. *J Neurosci* 20:7116-7121.

Mogenson GJ, Nielsen M (1984) A study of the contribution of hippocampal-accumbens-subpallidal projections to locomotor activity. *Behav Neural Biol* 42:38-51.

Molteni R, Ying Z, Gomez-Pinilla F (2002) Differential effects of acute and chronic exercise on plasticity-related genes in the rat hippocampus revealed by microarray. Eur J Neurosci 16:1107-1116.

Neeper SA, Gomez-Pinilla F, Choi J, Cotman C (1995) Exercise and brain neurotrophins. *Nature* 373:109.

Neeper SA, Gomez-Pinilla F, Choi J, Cotman CW (1996) Physical activity increases mRNA for brain-derived neurotrophic factor and nerve growth factor in rat brain. *Brain Res* 726:49-56.

Pelleymounter MA, Cullen MJ, Baker MB, Gollub M, Wellman C (1996) The effects of intrahippocampal BDNF and NGF on spatial learning in aged Long Evans rats. *Mol Chem Neuropathol* 29:211-226.

Peters A, Moss MB, Sethares C (2001) The effects of aging on layer 1 of primary visual cortex in the rhesus monkey. *Cereb Cortex* 11:93-103.

Peters A, Rosene DL, Moss MB, Kemper TL, Abraham CR, Tigges J, Albert MS (1996) Neurobiological bases of age-related cognitive decline in the rhesus monkey. *J Neuropathol Exp Neurol* 55:861-874.

Plaznik A, Stefanski R, Kostowski W (1990) GABAergic mechanisms in the nucleus accumbens septi regulating rat motor activity: the effect of chronic treatment with desipramine. *Pharmacol Biochem Behav* 36:501-506.

References

Poulton NP, Muir GD (2005) Treadmill training ameliorates dopamine loss but not behavioral deficits in hemi-parkinsonian rats. Exp Neurol 193:181-197.

Ramon Y Cajal S, Defelipe J, Jones EG (1988) Cajal on the cerebral cortex: an annotated translation of the complete writings. History of neuroscience, no. 1. New York, Oxford University Press.

Ramsden M, Berchtold NC, Patrick Kesslak J, Cotman CW, Pike CJ (2003) Exercise increases the vulnerability of rat hippocampal neurons to kainate lesion. *Brain Res* 971:239-244.

Rhodes JS, van Praag H, Jeffrey S, Girard I, Mitchell GS, Garland T, Jr., Gage FH (2003) Exercise increases hippocampal neurogenesis to high levels but does not improve spatial learning in mice bred for increased voluntary wheel running. *Behav Neurosci* 117:1006-1016.

Roland PE, Meyer E, Shibasaki T, Yamamoto YL, Thompson CJ (1982) Regional cerebral blood flow changes in cortex and basal ganglia during voluntary movements in normal human volunteers. *J Neurophysiol* 48:467-480.

Runquist EA, Heron WT (1935) Spontaneous activity and maze learning. *J Comp Psychol* 19:297-311.

Russo-Neustadt AA, Chen MJ (2005) Brain-derived neurotrophic factor and antidepressant activity. *Curr Pharm Des* 11:1495-1510.

Russo-Neustadt A, Ha T, Ramirez R, Kesslak JP (2001) Physical activity-antidepressant treatment combination: impact on brain-derived neurotrophic factor and behavior in an animal model. *Behav Brain Res* 120:87-95.

Rutledge LT, Wright C, Duncan J (1974) Morphological changes in pyramidal cells of mammalian neocortex associated with increased use. Exp Neurol 44:209-228.

Salat DH, Buckner RL, Snyder AZ, Greve DN, Desikan RS, Busa E, Morris JC, Dale AM, Fischl B (2004) Thinning of the cerebral cortex in aging. *Cereb Cortex* 14:721-730.

Samorajski T, Rolsten C (1975) Nerve fiber hypertrophy in posterior tibial nerves of mice in response to voluntary running activity during aging. *J Comp Neurol* 159:553-558.

Samorajski T, Rolsten C, Przykorska A, Davis CM (1987) Voluntary wheel running exercise and monoamine levels in brain, heart and adrenal glands of aging mice. *Exp Gerontol* 22:421-431.

Santarelli L, Saxe M, Gross C, Surget A, Battaglia F, Dulawa S, Weisstaub N, Lee J, Duman R, Arancio O, Belzung C, Hen R (2003) Requirement of hippocampal neurogenesis for the behavioral effects of antidepressants. *Science* 301:805-809.

Shi LH, Luo F, Woodward DJ, Chang JY (2004) Neural responses in multiple basal ganglia regions during spontaneous and treadmill locomotion tasks in rats. *Exp Brain Res* 157:303-314.

Shirley M (1928) Studies in activity IV: The relation of activity to maze learning and brain weight. *J Comp Psychol* 8:187-195.

References

Shors TJ, Townsend DA, Zhao M, Kozorovitskiy Y, Gould E (2002) Neurogenesis may relate to some but not all types of hippocampal-dependent learning. *Hippocampus* 12:578-584.

Skalicky M, Bubna-Littitz H, Viidik A (1996) Influence of physical exercise on aging rats: I. Life-long exercise preserves patterns of spontaneous activity. *Mech Ageing Dev* 87:127-139.

Skalicky M, Viidik A (1999) Comparison between continuous and intermittent physical exercise on aging rats: changes in patterns of spontaneous activity and connective tissue stability. *Aging (Milano)* 11:227-234.

Sothmann MS, Buckworth J, Claytor RP, Cox RH, White-Welkley JE, Dishman RK (1996) Exercise training and the cross-stressor adaptation hypothesis. *Exerc Sport Sci Rev* 24:267-287.

Spirduso WW, Farrar RP (1981) Effects of aerobic training on reactive capacity: an animal model. *J Gerontol* 36:654-662.

Stummer W, Weber K, Tranmer B, Baethmann A, Kempski O (1994) Reduced mortality and brain damage after locomotor activity in gerbil forebrain ischemia. *Stroke* 25:1862-1869.

Swain RA, Harris AB, Wiener EC, Dutka MV, Morris HD, Theien BE, Konda S, Engberg K, Lauterbur PC, Greenough WT (2003) Prolonged exercise induces angiogenesis and increases cerebral blood volume in primary motor cortex of the rat. *Neuroscience* 117:1037-1046.

Tanapat P, Hastings NB, Rydel TA, Galea LA, Gould E (2001) Exposure to fox odor inhibits cell proliferation in the hippocampus of adult rats via an adrenal hormone-dependent mechanism. *J Comp Neurol* 437:496-504.

Tanzi E (1893) I fatti e le induzioni nell'odierna istoliga del sistema nervoso. *Rev Sperim d Frenatria et d Medic Legal XIX*.

Tillerson JL, Caudle WM, Reveron ME, Miller GW (2003) Exercise induces behavioral recovery and attenuates neurochemical deficits in rodent models of Parkinson's disease. *Neuroscience* 119:899-911.

Tong L, Shen H, Perreau VM, Balazs R, Cotman CW (2001) Effects of exercise on gene-expression profile in the rat hippocampus. *Neurobiol Dis* 8:1046-1056.

Tousoulis D, Charakida M, Stefanadis C (2005) Inflammation and endothelial dysfunction as therapeutic targets in patients with heart failure. *Int J Cardiol* 100:347-353.

Vanderwolf CH (1988) Cerebral activity and behavior: control by central cholinergic and serotonergic systems. *Int Rev Neurobiol* 30:225-340.

Van Hoomissen JD, Holmes PV, Zellner AS, Poudevigne A, Dishman RK (2004) Effects of beta-adrenoreceptor blockade during chronic exercise on contextual fear conditioning and mRNA for galanin and brain-derived neurotrophic factor. *Behav Neurosci* 118:1378-1390.

van Praag H, Christie BR, Sejnowski TJ, Gage FH (1999a) Running enhances neurogenesis, learning, and long-term potentiation in mice. *Proc Natl Acad Sci USA* 96:13427-13431.

van Praag H, Kempermann G, Gage FH (1999b) Running increases cell proliferation and neurogenesis in the adult mouse dentate gyrus. *Nat Neurosci* 2:266-270.

Vaynman S, Ying Z, Gomez-Pinilla F (2004) Hippocampal BDNF mediates the efficacy of exercise on synaptic plasticity and cognition. *Eur J Neurosci* 20:2580-2590.

Vissing J, Andersen M, Diemer NH (1996) Exercise-induced changes in local cerebral glucose utilization in the rat. *J Cereb Blood Flow Metab* 16:729-736.

Vollmayr B, Simonis C, Weber S, Gass P, Henn F (2003) Reduced cell proliferation in the dentate gyrus is not correlated with the development of learned helplessness. Biol Psychiatry 54:1035-1040.

Wallace DG, Hines DJ, Whishaw IQ (2002) Quantification of a single exploratory trip reveals hippocampal formation mediated dead reckoning. *J Neurosci Meth* 113:131-145.

Wallace DG, Whishaw IQ (2003) NMDA lesions of Ammon's horn and the dentate gyrus disrupt the direct and temporally paced homing displayed by rats exploring a novel environment: evidence for a role of the hippocampus in dead reckoning. *Eur J Neurosci* 18:513-523.

Wallenstein GV, Eichenbaum H, Hasselmo ME (1998) The hippocampus as an associator of discontiguous events. *Trends Neurosci* 21:317-323.

White NM, McDonald RJ (2002) Multiple parallel memory systems in the brain of the rat. *Neurobiol Learn Mem* 77:125-184.

Chapter 6

Adleman, N.E., Menon, V., Blasey, C.M., White, C.D., Warsofsky, I.S., Glover, G.H., & Reiss, A.L. (2002). A developmental fMRI study of the Stroop Color-Word Task. *NeuroImage, 16,* 61-75.

Baddeley, A. (1996). Exploring the central executive. *Quarterly Journal of Experimental Psychology, 49A,* 5-28.

Bashore, T.R. (1989). Age, physical fitness, and mental processing speed. *Annual Review of Gerontology and Geriatrics, 9,* 120-144.

Bernstein, P.S., Scheffers, M.K., & Coles, M.G.H. (1995). "Where did I go wrong?" A psychophysiological analysis of error detection. *Journal of Experimental Psychology: Human Perception and Performance, 21,* 1312-1322.

Black, J.E., Isaacs, K.R., Anderson, B.J., Alcantara, A.A., & Greenough, W.T. (1990). Learning causes synaptogenesis, whereas motor activity causes angiogenesis, in cerebellar cortex of adult rats. *Proceedings of the National Academy of Science, 87,* 5568-5572.

Blomstrand, E., Perrett, D., Parry-Billings, M., & Newsholme, E.A. (1989). Effect of sustained exercise on plasma amino acid concentrations and on 5-hydroxytryptamine metabolism in six different brain regions in the rat. *Acta Physiologica Scandinavica, 136,* 473-481.

References

Botvinick, M.M., Braver, T.S., Barch, D.M., Carter, C.S., & Cohen, J.D. (2001). Conflict monitoring and cognitive control. *Psychological Review, 108,* 624-652.

Botvinick, M., Nystrom, L.E., Fissell, K., Carter, C.S., & Cohen, J.D. (1999). Conflict monitoring versus selection-for-action in anterior cingulated cortex. *Nature, 402,* 179-181.

Brozoski, T.J., Brown, R.M., Rosvold, H.E., & Goldman, P.S. (1979). Cognitive deficits caused by regional depletion of dopamine in prefrontal cortex of rhesus monkeys. *Science, 205,* 929-932.

Buck, S.M., Hillman, C.H., & Castelli, D.M. (2008). Aerobic fitness influences on Stroop task performance in healthy preadolescent children. *Medicine & Science in Sports & Exercise, 40,* 166-172.

Buckner, R.L., Head, D., & Lustig, C. (2006). Brain changes in aging. In E. Bialystok & F.I.M. Craik (Eds.), *Lifespan cognition: Mechanisms of change* (pp. 27-42). New York: Oxford University Press.

Bunge, S.A., Dudukovic, N.M., Thomason, M.E., Vaidya, C.J., & Gabrieli, J.D.E. (2002). Immature frontal lobe contributions to cognitive control in children: Evidence from fMRI. *Neuron, 33,* 301-311.

Carro, E., Trejo, J.L., Busiguina, S., & Torres-Aleman, I. (2001). Circulating insulin-like growth factor 1 mediates the protective effects of physical exercise against brain insults of different etiology and anatomy. *Journal of Neuroscience, 21,* 5678-5684.

Carter, C.S., Braver, T.S., Barch, D.M., Botvinick, M.M., Noll, D., & Cohen, J.D. (1998). Anterior cingulated cortex, error detection, and the online monitoring of performance. *Science, 280,* 747-749.

Carter, C.S., Macdonald, A.M., Botvinick, M., Ross, L.L., Stenger, V.A., Noll, D., & Cohen, J.D. (2000). Parsing executive processes: Strategic vs. evaluative functions of the anterior cingulate cortex. *Proceedings of the National Academy of Sciences, 97,* 1944-1948.

Castelli, D.M., Hillman, C.H., Buck, S.M., & Erwin, H. (2007). Physical fitness and academic achievement in 3rd & 5th grade students. *Journal of Sport and Exercise Psychology, 29,* 239-252.

Colcombe, S.J., & Kramer, A.F. (2003). Fitness effects on the cognitive function of older adults: A meta-analytic study. *Psychological Science, 14,* 125-130.

Colcombe, S.J., Kramer, A.F., Erickson, K.I., Scalf, P., McAuley, E., Cohen, N.J., Webb, A., et al. (2004). Cardiovascular fitness, cortical plasticity, and aging. *Proceedings of the National Academy of Sciences, 101,* 3316-3321.

Coles, M.G.H., & Rugg, M.D. (1995). Event-related potentials: An introduction. In M.D. Rugg & M.G.H. Coles (Eds.), *Electrophysiology of mind* (pp. 1-26). New York: Oxford University Press.

Cotman, C.W., & Berchtold, N.C. (2002). Exercise: A behavioral intervention to enhance brain health and plasticity. *Trends in Neurosciences, 25,* 295-301.

References

Davies, P.L., Segalowitz, S.J., Dywan, J., & Pailing, P.E. (2001). Error-negativity and positivity as they relate to other ERP indices of attentional control and stimulus processing. *Biological Psychology, 56,* 191-206.

Davis, P., & Wright, E.A. (1977). A new method for measuring cranial cavity volume and its application to the assessment of cerebral atrophy at autopsy. *Neuropathology and Applied Neurobiology, 3,* 341-358.

Dehaene, S., Posner, M.I., & Tucker, D.M. (1994). Localization of a neural system for error detection and compensation. *Psychological Science, 5,* 303-305.

Demetriou, A., Spanoudis, G., Christou, C., & Platsidou, M. (2002). Modeling the Stroop phenomenon: Processes, processing flow, and development. *Cognitive Development, 16,* 987-1005.

Dempster, F.N. (1992). The rise and fall of the inhibitory mechanism: Toward a unified theory of cognitive development and aging. *Developmental Review, 12,* 45-75.

Diamond, A. (2006). The early development of executive functions. In E. Bialystok & F.I.M. Craik (Eds.), *Lifespan cognition: Mechanisms of change* (pp. 70-95). New York: Oxford University Press.

Diamond, A., Towle, C., & Boyer, K. (1994). Young children's performance on a task sensitive to the memory functions of the medial temporal lobe in adults, the delayed nonmatching-to-sample task, reveals problems that are due to non-memory-related task demands. *Behavioral Neuroscience, 108,* 659-680.

DiPietro, L., Casperson, C.J., Ostfeld, A.M., & Nadel, E.R. (1993). A survey for assessing physical activity among older adults. *Medicine and Science in Sports and Exercise, 25,* 628-642.

Donchin, E. (1981). Surprise! . . . surprise? *Psychophysiology, 18,* 493-513.

Donchin, E., & Coles, M.G.H. (1988). Is the P3 component a manifestation of context updating? *Brain Behavioral Science, 11,* 357-374.

Duncan-Johnson, C.C. (1981). P3 latency: A new metric of information processing. *Psychophysiology, 18,* 207-215.

Dustman, R.E., Emmerson, R.Y., Ruhling, R.O., Shearer, D.E., Steinhaus, L.A., Johnson, S.C., et al. (1990). Age and fitness effects on EEG, ERPs, visual sensitivity, and cognition. *Neurobiology of Aging, 11,* 193-200.

Dustman, R.E., LaMarsh, J.A., Cohn, N.B., Shearer, D.E., & Talone, J.M. (1985). Power spectral analysis and cortical coupling of EEG for young and old normal adults. *Neurobiology of Aging, 6,* 193-198.

Dustman, R.E., Shearer, D.E., & Emmerson, R.E. (1993). EEG and event-related potentials in normal aging. *Progress in Neurobiology, 41,* 369-401.

Eriksen, B.A., & Eriksen, C.W. (1974). Effects of noise letters upon the identification of a target letter in a nonsearch task. *Perception & Psychophysics, 16,* 143-149.

Eriksen, C.W., & Schultz, D.W. (1979). Information processing in visual search: A continuous flow conception and experimental results. *Perception and Psychophysics, 25,* 249-263.

References

Fabiani, M., & Friedman, D. (1995). Changes in brain activity patterns in aging: The novelty oddball. *Psychophysiology, 32,* 579-594.

Fabiani, M., Friedman, D., & Cheng, J.C. (1998). Individual differences in P3 scalp distribution in older adults, and their relationship to frontal lobe function. *Psychophysiology, 35,* 698-708.

Falkenstein, M., Hohnsbein, J., Hoormann, J., & Blanke, L. (1990). Effects of errors in choice reaction tasks on the ERP under focused and divided attention. In C.H.M. Brunia, A.W.K. Gaillard, & A. Kok (Eds.), *Psychophysiological brain research* (Vol. 1, pp. 192-195). Tilberg, The Netherlands: Tilberg University Press.

Falkenstein, M., Hohnsbein, J., Hoormann, J., & Blanke, L. (1991). Effects of crossmodal divided attention on late ERP components: II. Error processing in choice reaction tasks. *Electroencephalography and Clinical Neurophysiology, 78,* 447-455.

Falkenstein, M., Hoormann, J., Christ, S., & Hohnsbein, J. (2000). ERP components on reaction errors and their functional significance: A tutorial. *Biological Psychology, 51,* 87-107.

Farrell, P.A., Gustafson, A.B., Garthwaite, T.L., Kalkhoff, R.K., Cowley Jr., A.W., & Morgan, W.P. (1986). Influence of endogenous opioids on the response of selected hormones to exercise in humans. *Journal of Applied Physiology, 61,* 1051-1057.

Fotenos, A.F., Snyder, A.Z., Girton, L.E., Morris, J.C., & Buckner, R.L. (2005). Normative estimates of cross-sectional and longitudinal brain volume decline in aging and AD. *Neurology, 64,* 1032-1039.

Friedman, D., Simpson, G., & Hamberger, M. (1993). Age-related changes in scalp topography to novel and target stimuli. *Psychophysiology, 30,* 383-396.

Gehring, W.J., Goss, B., Coles, M.G.H., Meyer, D.E., & Donchin, E. (1993). A neural system for error detection and compensation. *Psychological Science, 4,* 385-390.

Gehring, W.J., & Knight, R.T. (2000). Prefrontal-cingulate interactions in action monitoring. *Nature Neuroscience, 3,* 516-520.

Gonsalvez, C.J., & Polich, J. (2002). P3 amplitude is determined by target-to-target interval. *Psychophysiology, 39,* 388-396.

Gullestad, L., Myers, J., Bjornerheim, R., Berg, K.J., Djoseland, O., Hall, C., Lund, K., Kjekshus, J., & Simonsen, S. (1997). Gas exchange and neurohumoral response to exercise: Influence of the exercise protocol. *Medicine and Science in Sports and Exercise, 29,* 496-502.

Hasher, L., & Zachs, R.T. (1988). Working memory, comprehension, and aging: A review and a new view. In G.H. Bower (Ed.), *The psychology of learning and motivation* (Vol. 22, pp. 193-225). New York: Academic Press.

Hatta, A., Nishihira, Y., Kim, S.R., Kaneda, T., Kida, T., Kamijo, K., Sasahara, M., & Haga, S. (2005). Effects of habitual moderate exercise on response processing and cognitive processing in older adults. *Japanese Journal of Physiology, 55,* 29-36.

References

Haug, H., & Eggers, R. (1991). Morphometry of the human cortex cerebri and corpus striatum during aging. *Neurobiology of Aging, 12,* 336-338.

Herrmann, M.J., Römmler, J., Ehlis, A., Heidrich, A., & Fallgatter, A.J. (2004). Source localization (LORETA) of the error-related-negativity (ERN/Ne) and positivity (Pe). *Cognitive Brain Research, 20,* 294-299.

Hillman, C.H., Belopolsky, A., Snook, E.M., Kramer, A.F., & McAuley, E. (2004). Physical activity and executive control: Implications for increased cognitive health during older adulthood. *Research Quarterly for Exercise and Sport, 75,* 176-185.

Hillman, C.H., Buck, S.M., Themanson, J.T., Pontifex, M.B., & Castelli, D.M. (in press). Aerobic fitness and cognitive development: Event-related brain potential and task performance indices of executive control in preadolescent children. *Developmental Psychology.*

Hillman, C.H., Castelli, D.M., & Buck, S.M. (2005). Aerobic fitness and neurocognitive function in healthy preadolescent children. *Medicine and Science in Sports and Exercise, 37,* 1967-1974.

Hillman, C.H., Kramer, A.F., Belopolsky, A.V., & Smith, D.P. (2006). A cross-sectional examination of age and physical activity on performance and event-related brain potentials in a task switching paradigm. *International Journal of Psychophysiology, 59,* 30-39.

Hillman, C.H., Snook, E.M., & Jerome, G.J. (2003). Acute cardiovascular exercise and executive control function. *International Journal of Psychophysiology, 48,* 307-314.

Hillman, C.H., Weiss, E.P., Hagberg, J.M., & Hatfield, B.D. (2002). The relationship of age and cardiovascular fitness to cognitive and motor processes. *Psychophysiology, 39,* 303-312.

Holroyd, C.B., & Coles, M.G.H. (2002). The neural basis of human error processing: Reinforcement learning, dopamine, and the error-related negativity. *Psychological Review, 109,* 679-709.

Hugdahl, K. (1995). *Psychophysiology: The mind-body perspective.* Cambridge, MA: Harvard University Press.

Isaacs, K.R., Anderson, B.J., Alcantara, A.A., Black, J.E., & Greenough, W.T. (1992). Exercise and the brain: Angiogenesis in the adult rat cerebellum after vigorous physical activity and motor skill learning. *Journal of Cerebral Blood Flow and Metabolism, 12,* 110-119.

Kerns, J.G., Cohen, J.D., MacDonald, A.W. III, Cho, R.Y., Stenger, V.A., & Carter, C.S. (2004). Anterior cingulate conflict monitoring and adjustments in control. *Science, 303,* 1023-1026.

Klenberg, L., Korkman, M., & Lahti-Nuuttila, P. (2001). Differential development of attention and executive functions in 3-12 year old Finnish children. *Developmental Neuropsychology, 20,* 407-428.

Knight, R.T. (1984). Decreased response to novel stimuli after prefrontal lesions in man. *Electroencephalography and Clinical Neurophysiology, 52,* 9-20.

Knight, R.T. (1996). Contributions of human hippocampal region to novelty detection. *Nature, 383,* 256-259.

Knight, R.T. (1997). Distributed cortical network for visual attention. *Journal of Cognitive Neuroscience, 9,* 75-91.

Kramer, A.F., Colcombe, S.J., McAuley, E., Scalf, P.E., & Erickson, K.I. (2005). Fitness, aging, and neurocognitive function. *Neurobiology of Aging, 26,* 124-127.

Kramer, A.F., Hahn, S., & Gopher, D. (1999). Task coordination and aging: Explorations of executive control processes in the task switching paradigm. *Acta Physiologica Scandinavica, 101,* 339-378.

Kramer, A.F., & Hillman, C.H. (2006). Aging, physical activity, and neurocognitive function. In E. Acevedo & P. Ekkekakis (Eds.), *Psychobiology of physical activity* (pp. 45-59). Champaign, IL: Human Kinetics.

Kramer, A.F., Humphrey, D.G., Larish, J.F., Logan, G.B., & Strayer, D.L. (1994). Aging and inhibition: Beyond a unitary view of inhibitory processing in attention. *Psychology and Aging, 9,* 491-512.

Kramer, A.F., & Kray, J. (2006). Aging and attention. In E. Bialystok & F.I.M. Craik (Eds.), *Lifespan cognition: Mechanisms of change* (pp. 57-69). New York: Oxford University Press.

Kramer, A.F., Sowon, H., Cohen, N.J., Banich, M.T., McAuley, E., Harrison, C.R., Chason, J., Vakil, E., Bardell, L., Boileau, R.A., & Colcombe, A. (1999). Ageing, fitness, and neurocognitive function. *Nature, 400,* 418-419.

Luciana, M., & Nelson, C.A. (1998). The functional emergence of prefrontally-guided working memory systems in four- to eight-year-old children. *Neuropsychologia, 36,* 273-293.

Luck, S.J. (2005). *An introduction to the event-related potential technique.* Cambridge, MA: MIT Press.

Luria, A.R. (1973). *The working brain: An introduction to neuropsychology.* New York: Basic Books.

MacDonald, A.W., Cohen, J.D., Stenger, V.A., & Carter, C.S. (2000). Dissociating the role of dorsolateral prefrontal and anterior cingulate cortex in cognitive control. *Science, 288,* 1835-1838.

MacLeod, C.M. (1991). Half a century of research on the Stroop effect: An integrative review. *Psychological Bulletin, 109,* 163-203.

MacRae, P.G., Spirduso, W.W., Cartee, G.D., Farrar, R.P., & Wilcox, R.E. (1987). Endurance training effects on striatal D_2 dopamine receptor binding and striatal dopamine metabolite levels. *Neuroscience Letters, 79,* 138-144.

Mathewson, K.J., Dywan, J., & Segalowitz, S.J. (2005). Brain bases of error-related ERPs as influenced by age and task. *Biological Psychology, 70,* 88-104.

McDowell, K., Kerick, S.E., Santa Maria, D.L., & Hatfield, B.D. (2003). Aging, physical activity, and cognitive processing: An examination of P300. *Neurobiology of Aging, 24,* 597-606.

References

Meeusen, R., Smolders, I., Sarre, S., De Meirleir, K., Keizer, H., Serneels, M., Ebinger, G., & Michotte, Y. (1997). Endurance training effects on neurotransmitter release in rat striatum: An in vivo microdialysis study. *Acta Physiologica Scandinavica, 159,* 335-341.

Meyer, D.E., & Kieras, D.E. (1997). A computational theory of executive cognitive processes and multi-task performance: Part 1. Basic mechanisms. *Psychological Review, 104,* 3-65.

Miltner, W.H.R., Lemke, U., Weiss, T., Holroyd, C., Scheffers, M.K., & Coles, M.G.H. (2003). Implementation of error-processing in the human anterior cingulated cortex: A source analysis of the magnetic equivalent of the error-related negativity. *Biological Psychology, 64,* 157-166.

Miyake, A., Friedman, N.P., Emerson, M.J., Witzki, A.H., & Howerter, A. (2000). The unity and diversity of executive functions and their contributions to complex "frontal lobe" tasks: A latent variable analysis. *Cognitive Psychology, 41,* 49-100.

Neeper, S.A., Gómez-Pinilla, F., Choi, J., & Cotman, C. (1995). Exercise and brain neurotrophins. *Nature, 373,* 109.

Nieuwenhuis, S., Ridderinkhof, K.R., Blom, J., Band, G.P.H., & Kok, A. (2001). Error-related brain potentials are differentially related to awareness of response errors: Evidence from an antisaccade task. *Psychophysiology, 38,* 752-760.

Norman, D.A., & Shallice, T. (1986). Attention to action: Willed and automatic control of behavior. In R.J. Davidson, G.E. Schwartz, & D. Shapiro (Eds.), *Consciousness and self-regulation:* Vol. 4. *Advances in research and theory* (pp. 1-18). New York: Plenum Press.

O'Donnell, B.F., Friedman, S., Swearer, J.M., & Drachman, D.A. (1992). Active and passive P3 latency and psychometric performance: Influence of age and individual differences. *International Journal of Psychophysiology, 12,* 187-195.

Park, D.C., Lautenschlager, G., Hedden, T., Davidson, N.S., Smith, A.D., & Smith, P.K. (2002). Models of visuospatial and verbal memory across the adult life span. *Psychology and Aging, 17,* 299-320.

Parnpiansil, P., Jutapakdeegul, N., Chentanez, T., & Kotchabhakdi, N. (2003). Exercise during pregnancy increases hippocampal brain-derived neurotrophic factor mRNA expression and spatial learning in neonatal rat pup. *Neuroscience Letters, 352,* 45-48.

Picton, T.W., Stuss, D.T., Champagne, S.C., & Nelson, R.F. (1984). The effects of age on human event-related potentials. *Psychophysiology, 21,* 312-325.

Polich, J. (1997). EEG and ERP assessment of normal aging. *Electroencephalography and Clinical Neurophysiology, 104,* 244-256.

Polich, J. (2004). Clinical applications of the P300 event-related brain potential. *Physical Medicine and Rehabilitation Clinics of North America, 15,* 133-161.

Polich, J., & Heine, M.R.D. (1996). P3 topography and modality effects from a single-stimulus paradigm. *Psychophysiology, 33,* 747-752.

References

Polich, J., & Lardon, M. (1997). P300 and long term physical exercise. *Electroencephalography and Clinical Neurophysiology, 103,* 493-498.

Posner, M.I. (1992). Attention as a cognitive neural system. *Current Directions in Psychological Science, 1,* 11-14.

Posner, M.I., & Petersen, S.E. (1990). The attention system of the human brain. *Annual Review of Neuroscience, 13,* 25-42.

Rabbitt, P.M.A. (1966). Error correction time without external error signals. *Nature, 212,* 438.

Rabbitt, P.M.A. (2002). Consciousness is slower than you think. *Quarterly Journal of Experimental Psychology, 55A,* 1081-1092.

Rabbitt, P.M.A., Cumming, G., & Vyas, S.M. (1978). Some errors of perceptual analysis in visual search can be detected and corrected. *Quarterly Journal of Experimental Psychology, 30,* 319-332.

Raz, N. (2000). Aging of the brain and its impact on cognitive performance: Integration of structural and functional findings. In F.I.M. Craik & T.A. Salthouse (Eds.), *The handbook of aging and cognition* (2nd ed., pp. 1-90). Mahwah, NJ: Erlbaum.

Rhyu, I.J., Boklewski, J., Ferguson, B., Lee, K., Lange, H., Bytheway, J., Lamb, J., McCormick, K., Williams, N., Cameron, J., & Greenough, W.T. (2003). Exercise training associated with increased cortical vascularization in adult female cynomologus monkeys. *Society for Neuroscience Abstracts, 920,* 1.

Robbins, T.W., James, M., Owen, A.M., Shaakian, B.J., Lawrence, A.D., McInnes, L., & Rabbit, P.M.A. (1998). A study of performance from tests from the CANTAB battery sensitive to frontal lobe dysfunction in a large sample of normal volunteers: Implications for theories of executive functioning and cognitive aging. *Journal of the International Neuropsychological Society, 4,* 474-490.

Rogers, R.D., & Monsell, S. (1995). Costs of a predictable switch between simple cognitive tasks. *Journal of Experimental Psychology: General, 124,* 207-231.

Rueda, M.R., Fan, J., McCandliss, B.D., Halparin, J.D., Gruber, D.B., Lercari, L.P., & Posner, M.I. (2004). Development of attentional networks in childhood. *Neuropsychologia, 42,* 1029-1040.

Salat, D.H., Buckner, R.L., Snyder, A.Z., Greve, D.N., Desikan, R.S., Busa, E., et al. (2004). Thinning of the cerebral cortex in aging. *Cerebral Cortex, 14,* 721-730.

Scheffers, M.K., Coles, M.G.H., Bernstein, P., Gehring, W.J., & Donchin, E. (1996). Event-related brain potentials and error-related processing: An analysis of incorrect responses to go and no-go stimuli. *Psychophysiology, 33,* 42-53.

Schretlen, D., Pearlson, G.D., Anthony, J.C., Aylward, E.H., Augustine, A.M., Davis, A., & Barta, P. (2000). Elucidating the contributions of processing speed, executive ability, and frontal lobe volume to normal age-related differences in fluid intelligence. *Journal of the International Neuropsychological Society, 6,* 52-61.

Sibley, B.A., & Etnier, J.L. (2003). The relationship between physical activity and cognition in children: A meta-analysis. *Pediatric Exercise Science, 15,* 243-256.

References

Siegler, R.S. (1998). *Children's thinking.* Upper Saddle River, NJ: Prentice Hall.

Spencer, K.M., & Coles, M.G.H. (1999). The lateralized readiness potential: Relationship between human data and response activation in a connectionist model. *Psychophysiology, 36,* 364-370.

Spirduso, W.W., & Farrar, R.P. (1981). Effects of aerobic training on reactive capacity: An animal model. *Journal of Gerontology, 35,* 654-662.

Squire, L.R., & Kandell, E.R. (1999). *Memory from mind to molecules.* New York: Scientific American Library.

Sutton, S., Braren, M., Zubin, J., & John, E.R. (1965). Evoked potential correlates of stimulus uncertainty. *Science, 150,* 1187-1188.

Swain, R.A., Harris, A.B., Wiener, E.C., Dutka, M.V., Morris, H.D., Theien, B.E., Konda, S., Engberg, K., Lauterbur, P.C., & Greenough, W.T. (2003). Prolonged exercise induces angiogenesis and increases cerebral blood volume in primary motor cortex of the rat. *Neuroscience, 117,* 1037-1046.

Tekok-Kilic, A., Shucard, J.L., & Shucard, D.W. (2001). Stimulus modality and Go/NoGo effects on P3 during parallel visual and auditory continuous performance tasks. *Psychophysiology, 38,* 578-589.

Themanson, J.R., & Hillman, C.H. (2006). Cardiorespiratory fitness and acute aerobic exercise effects on neuroelectric and behavioral measures of action monitoring. *Neuroscience, 141,* 757-767.

Themanson, J.R., Hillman, C.H., & Curtin, J.J. (2006). Age and physical activity influences on neuroelectric indices of action monitoring during task switching. *Neurobiology of Aging, 27,* 1335-1345.

Van Loon, G.R., Schwartz, L., & Sole, M.J. (1979). Plasma dopamine response to standing and exercise in man. *Life Sciences, 24,* 2273-2278.

van Veen, V., & Carter, C.S. (2002). The timing of action-monitoring processes in the anterior cingulated cortex. *Journal of Cognitive Neuroscience, 14,* 593-602.

Wang, G.J., Volkow, N.D., Fowler, J.S., Franceschi, D., Logan, J., Pappas, N.R., Wong, C.T., & Netusil, N. (2000). PET studies of the effects of aerobic exercise on human striatal dopamine release. *Journal of Nuclear Medicine, 41,* 1352-1356.

Welk, G.J., Morrow, J.R.J., & Falls, H.B. (2002). *Fitnessgram reference guide.* Dallas: Cooper Institute.

West, R.L. (1996). An application of prefrontal cortex function theory to cognitive aging. *Psychological Bulletin, 120,* 272-292.

Yeung, N., Cohen, J.D., & Botvinick, M.M. (2004). The neural basis of error detection: Conflict monitoring and the error-related negativity. *Psychological Review, 111,* 931-959.

Young, D.R., Jee, S.H., & Appel, L.J. (2001). A comparison of the Yale Physical Activity Survey with other physical activity measures. *Medicine and Science in Sports and Exercise, 33,* 955-961.

Zacks, R.T., & Hasher, L. (2006). Aging and long-term memory: Deficits are not inevitable. In E. Bialystok & F.I.M. Craik (Eds.), *Lifespan cognition: Mechanisms of change* (pp. 162-177). New York: Oxford University Press.

Zeef, E.J., Sonke, C.J., Kok, A., Buiten, M.M., & Kenemans, J.L. (1996). Perceptual factors affecting age-related differences in focused attention: Performance and psychophysiological analyses. *Psychophysiology, 33,* 555-565.

Zelazo, P.D., Craik, F.I.M., & Booth, L. (2004). Executive function across the life span. *Acta Psychologica, 115,* 167-183.

Chapter 7

Biacabe, B., Chevallier, J.M., Avan, P., & Bonfils, P. (2001). Functional anatomy of auditory brainstem nuclei: application to the anatomical basis of brainstem auditory evoked potentials. *Auris, Nasus, Larynx, 28,* 85-94.

Bokura, H., Yamaguchi, S., & Kobayashi, S. (2001). Electrophysiological correlates for response inhibition in a Go/NoGo task. *Clinical Neurophysiology, 112,* 2224-2232.

Bruin, K.J., Wijers, A.A., & van Staveren, A.S. (2001). Response priming in a go/nogo task: do we have to explain the go/nogo N2 effect in terms of response activation instead of inhibition? *Clinical Neurophysiology, 112,* 1660-1671.

Carter, C.S., Macdonald, A.M., Botvinick, M., Ross, L.L., Stenger, V.A., Noll, D., et al. (2000). Parsing executive processes: strategic vs. evaluative functions of the anterior cingulate cortex. *Proceedings of the National Academy of Sciences USA, 97,* 1944-1948.

Chmura, J., Krysztofiak, H., Ziemba, A.W., Nazar, K., & Kaciuba-Uscilko, H. (1998). Psychomotor performance during prolonged exercise above and below the blood lactate threshold. *European Journal of Applied Physiology and Occupational Physiology, 77,* 77-80.

Chmura, J., Nazar, K., & Kaciuba-Uscilko, H. (1994). Choice reaction time during graded exercise in relation to blood lactate and plasma catecholamine thresholds. *International Journal of Sports Medicine, 15,* 172-176.

Chodzko-Zajko, W.J. (1991). Physical fitness, cognitive performance, and aging. *Medicine and Science in Sports and Exercise, 23,* 868-872.

Chwilla, D.J., & Brunia, C.H. (1991). Event-related potentials to different feedback stimuli. *Psychophysiology, 28,* 123-132.

Collardeau, M., Brisswalter, J., Vercruyssen, F., Audiffren, M., & Goubault, C. (2001). Single and choice reaction time during prolonged exercise in trained subjects: influence of carbohydrate availability. *European Journal of Applied Physiology and Occupational Physiology, 86,* 150-156.

Crowley, K.E., & Colrain, I.M. (2004). A review of the evidence for P2 being an independent component process: age, sleep and modality. *Clinical Neurophysiology, 115,* 732-744.

References

Davies, P.L., Segalowitz, S.J., Dywan, J., & Pailing, P.E. (2001). Error-negativity and positivity as they relate to other ERP indices of attentional control and stimulus processing. *Biological Psychology, 56,* 191-206.

Donchin, E., & Coles, M.G.H. (1988). Is the P300 component a manifestation of context updating? *Behavioral and Brain Sciences, 11,* 357-427.

Duzova, H., Ozisik, H.I., Polat, A., Emre, M.H., & Gullu, E. (2005). Correlations between event-related potential components and nitric oxide in maximal anaerobic exercise among sportsmen trained at various levels. *International Journal of Neuroscience, 115,* 1353-1373.

Emery, C.F., Honn, V.J., Frid, D.J., Lebowitz, K.R., & Diaz, P.T. (2001). Acute effects of exercise on cognition in patients with chronic obstructive pulmonary disease. *American Journal of Respiratory and Critical Care Medicine, 164,* 1624-1627.

Eriksen, C.W., & Eriksen, B.A. (1974). Effects of noise letters upon the identification letter in a non-search task. *Perception and Psychophysics, 16,* 143-149.

Eriksen, C.W., & Schultz, D.W. (1979). Information processing in visual search: a continuous flow conception and experimental results. *Perception and Psychophysics, 25,* 249-263.

Falkenstein, M., Hoormann, J., Christ, S., & Hohnsbein, J. (2000). ERP components on reaction errors and their functional significance: a tutorial. *Biological Psychology, 51,* 87-107.

Falkenstein, M., Hoormann, J., & Hohnsbein, J. (1999). ERP components in Go/Nogo tasks and their relation to inhibition. *Acta Psychologica, 101,* 267-291.

Fallgatter, A.J., & Strik, W.K. (1999). The NoGo-anteriorization as a neurophysiological standard-index for cognitive response control. *International Journal of Psychophysiology, 32,* 233-238.

Funahashi, S. (2001). Neuronal mechanisms of executive control by the prefrontal cortex. *Neuroscience Research, 39,* 147-165.

Geisler, M.W., & Polich, J. (1990). P300 and time of day: circadian rhythms, food intake, and body temperature. *Biological Psychology, 31,* 117-136.

Grego, F., Vallier, J.M., Collardeau, M., Bermon, S., Ferrari, P., Candito, M., et al. (2004). Effects of long duration exercise on cognitive function, blood glucose, and counterregulatory hormones in male cyclists. *Neuroscience Letters, 364,* 76-80.

Gutin, B., & DiGennaro, J. (1968a). Effect of a treadmill run to exhaustion on performance of long addition. *Research Quarterly, 39,* 958-964.

Gutin, B., & DiGennaro, J. (1968b). Effect of one-minute and five-minute step-ups on performance of simple addition. *Research Quarterly, 39,* 81-85.

Hatta, A., Nishihira, Y., Kim, S.R., Kaneda, T., Kida, T., Kamijo, K., et al. (2005). Effects of habitual moderate exercise on response processing and cognitive processing in older adults. *Japanese Journal of Physiology, 55,* 29-36.

Higuchi, S., Watanuki, S., & Yasukouchi, A. (1997). Effects of reduction in arousal level caused by long-lasting task on CNV. *Applied Human Science, 16,* 29-34.

Higuchi, S., Watanuki, S., Yasukouchi, A., & Sato, M. (1997). Effects of changes in arousal level by continuous light stimulus on contingent negative variation (CNV). *Applied Human Science, 16,* 55-60.

Hillman, C.H., Belopolsky, A.V., Snook, E.M., Kramer, A.F., & McAuley, E. (2004). Physical activity and executive control: implications for increased cognitive health during older adulthood. *Research Quarterly for Exercise and Sport, 75,* 176-185.

Hillman, C.H., Kramer, A.F., Belopolsky, A.V., & Smith, D.P. (2006). A cross-sectional examination of age and physical activity on performance and event-related brain potentials in a task switching paradigm. *International Journal of Psychophysiology, 59,* 30-39.

Hillman, C.H., Snook, E.M., & Jerome, G.J. (2003). Acute cardiovascular exercise and executive control function. *International Journal of Psychophysiology, 48,* 307-314.

Hillman, C.H., Weiss, E.P., Hagberg, J.M., & Hatfield, B.D. (2002). The relationship of age and cardiovascular fitness to cognitive and motor processes. *Psychophysiology, 39,* 303-312.

Holroyd, C.B., & Coles, M.G. (2002). The neural basis of human error processing: reinforcement learning, dopamine, and the error-related negativity. *Psychological Review, 109,* 679-709.

Hruby, T., & Marsalek, P. (2003). Event-related potentials—the P3 wave. *Acta Neurobiologiae Experimentalis, 63,* 55-63.

Irwin, D.A., Knott, J.R., McAdam, D.W., & Rebert, C.S. (1966). Motivational determinants of the "contingent negative variation." *Electroencephalography and Clinical Neurophysiology, 21,* 538-543.

Kamijo, K., Nishihira, Y., Hatta, A., Kaneda, T., Kida, T., Higashiura, T., et al. (2004a). Changes in arousal level by differential exercise intensity. *Clinical Neurophysiology, 115,* 2693-2698.

Kamijo, K., Nishihira, Y., Hatta, A., Kaneda, T., Wasaka, T., Kida, T., et al. (2004b). Differential influences of exercise intensity on information processing in the central nervous system. *European Journal of Applied Physiology and Occupational Physiology, 92,* 305-311.

Kida, T., Nishihira, Y., Hatta, A., Wasaka, T., Tazoe, T., Sakajiri, Y., et al. (2004). Resource allocation and somatosensory P300 amplitude during dual task: effects of tracking speed and predictability of tracking direction. *Clinical Neurophysiology, 115,* 2616-2628.

Kjaer, M. (1989). Epinephrine and some other hormonal responses to exercise in man: with special reference to physical training. *International Journal of Sports Medicine, 10,* 2-15.

References

Kjaer, M., Farrell, P.A., Christensen, N.J., & Galbo, H. (1986). Increased epinephrine response and inaccurate glucoregulation in exercising athletes. *Journal of Applied Physiology, 61,* 1693-1700.

Kopp, B., Rist, F., & Mattler, U. (1996). N200 in the flanker task as a neurobehavioral tool for investigating executive control. *Psychophysiology, 33,* 282-294.

Kramer, A.F., & Hillman, C.H. (2006). Aging, physical activity, and neurocognitive function. In E. Acevedo & P. Ekkekakis (Eds.), *Psychobiology of Physical Activity* (pp. 45-59). Champaign, IL: Human Kinetics.

Kramer, A.F., Humphrey, D.G., Larish, J.F., Logan, G.D., & Strayer, D.L. (1994). Aging and inhibition: beyond a unitary view of inhibitory processing in attention. *Psychology and Aging, 9,* 491-512.

Kramer, A.F., & Jacobson, A. (1991). Perceptual organization and focused attention: the role of objects and proximity in visual processing. *Perception and Psychophysics, 50,* 267-284.

Kutas, M., & Federmeier, K.D. (2000). Electrophysiology reveals semantic memory use in language comprehension. *Trends in Cognitive Sciences, 4,* 463-470.

Lew, G.S., & Polich, J. (1993). P300, habituation, and response mode. *Physiology and Behavior, 53,* 111-117.

Loveless, N.E., & Sanford, A.J. (1974). Slow potential correlates of preparatory set. *Biological Psychology, 1,* 303-314.

Magnié, M.N., Bermon, S., Martin, F., Madany-Lounis, M., Gastaud, M., & Dolisi, C. (1998). Visual and brainstem auditory evoked potentials and maximal aerobic exercise: does the influence of exercise persist after body temperature recovery? *International Journal of Sports Medicine, 19,* 255-259.

Magnié, M.N., Bermon, S., Martin, F., Madany-Lounis, M., Suisse, G., Muhammad, W., et al. (2000). P300, N400, aerobic fitness, and maximal aerobic exercise. *Psychophysiology, 37,* 369-377.

Mathewson, K.J., Dywan, J., & Segalowitz, S.J. (2005). Brain bases of error related ERPs as influenced by age and task. *Biological Psychology, 70,* 88-104.

McCallum, W.C., Papakostopoulos, D., Gombi, R., Winter, A.L., Cooper, R., & Griffith, H.B. (1973). Event related slow potential changes in human brain stem. *Nature, 242,* 465-467.

McCarthy, G., & Donchin, E. (1981). A metric for thought: a comparison of P300 latency and reaction time. *Science, 211,* 77-80.

McMorris, T., & Graydon, J. (2000). The effect of incremental exercise on cognitive performance. *International Journal of Sport Psychology, 31,* 66-81.

Meyer, D.E., & Kieras, D.E. (1997). A computational theory of executive cognitive processes and multiple-task performance: part 1. Basic mechanisms. *Psychological Review, 104,* 3-65.

Molloy, D.W., Beerschoten, D.A., Borrie, M.J., Crilly, R.G., & Cape, R.D. (1988). Acute effects of exercise on neuropsychological function in elderly subjects. *Journal of the American Geriatrics Society, 36,* 29-33.

Näätänen, R. (1990). The role of attention in auditory information processing as revealed by event-related potentials and other brain measures of cognitive function. *Behavioral Brain Sciences, 13,* 201-288.

Nakamura, Y., Nishimoto, K., Akamatu, M., Takahashi, M., & Maruyama, A. (1999). The effect of jogging on P300 event related potentials. *Electromyography and Clinical Neurophysiology, 39,* 71-74.

Nielsen, B., Hyldig, T., Bidstrup, F., Gonzalez-Alonso, J., & Christoffersen, G.R. (2001). Brain activity and fatigue during prolonged exercise in the heat. *Pflugers Archive European Journal of Physiology, 442,* 41-48.

Norman, D.A., & Shallice, T. (1986). Attention to action: willed and automatic control of behavior. In R.J. Davidson, G.E. Schwartz, & D. Shapiro (Eds.), *Consciousness and self-regulation* (pp. 1-18). New York: Plenum Press.

Ozmerdivenli, R., Bulut, S., Bayar, H., Karacabey, K., Ciloglu, F., Peker, I., et al. (2005). Effects of exercise on visual evoked potentials. *International Journal of Neuroscience, 115,* 1043-1050.

Perner, J., & Lang, B. (1999). Development of theory of mind and executive control. *Trends in Cognitive Sciences, 3,* 337-344.

Pfefferbaum, A., Ford, J., Johnson, R., Jr., Wenegrat, B., & Kopell, B.S. (1983). Manipulation of P3 latency: speed vs. accuracy instructions. *Electroencephalography and Clinical Neurophysiology, 55,* 188-197.

Picton, T.W., Bentin, S., Berg, P., Donchin, E., Hillyard, S.A., Johnson, R., Jr., et al. (2000). Guidelines for using human event-related potentials to study cognition: recording standards and publication criteria. *Psychophysiology, 37,* 127-152.

Picton, T.W., & Low, M.D. (1971). The CNV and semantic content of stimuli in the experimental paradigm: effects of feedback. *Electroencephalography and Clinical Neurophysiology, 31,* 451-456.

Polich, J., & Kok, A. (1995). Cognitive and biological determinants of P300: an integrative review. *Biological Psychology, 41,* 103-146.

Pontifex, M.B., & Hillman, C.H. (2007). Neuroelectric and behavioral indices of interference control during acute cycling. *Clinical Neurophysiology, 118,* 570-580.

Ravden, D., & Polich, J. (1998). Habituation of P300 from visual stimuli. *International Journal of Psychophysiology, 30,* 359-365.

Schubert, M., Johannes, S., Koch, M., Wieringa, B.M., Dengler, R., & Munte, T.F. (1998). Differential effects of two motor tasks on ERPs in an auditory classification task: evidence of shared cognitive resources. *Neuroscience Research, 30,* 125-134.

Sjoberg, H. (1980). Physical fitness and mental performance during and after work. *Ergonomics, 23,* 977-985.

Stones, M.J., & Dawe, D. (1993). Acute exercise facilitates semantically cued memory in nursing home residents. *Journal of the American Geriatrics Society, 41,* 531-534.

Tecce, J.J. (1972). Contingent negative variation (CNV) and psychological processes in man. *Psychological Bulletin, 77,* 73-108.

References

Tecce, J.J., Savignano-Bowman, J., & Meinbresse, D. (1976). Contingent negative variation and the distraction-arousal hypothesis. *Electroencephalography and Clinical Neurophysiology, 41,* 277-286.

Themanson, J.R., & Hillman, C.H. (2006). Cardiorespiratory fitness and acute aerobic exercise effects on neuroelectric and behavioral measures of action monitoring. *Neuroscience, 141,* 757-767.

Thomas, C.J., Jones, J.D., Scott, P.D., & Rosenberg, M.E. (1991). The influence of exercise-induced temperature elevations on the auditory brain-stem response (ABR). *Clinical Otolaryngology and Allied Sciences, 16,* 138-141.

Tomporowski, P.D. (2003). Effects of acute bouts of exercise on cognition. *Acta Psychologica, 112,* 297-324.

Tomporowski, P.D., & Ellis, N.R. (1986). Effects of exercise on cognitive processes: a review. *Psychological Bulletin, 99,* 338-346.

Tomporowski, P.D., Ellis, N.R., & Stephens, R. (1987). The immediate effects of strenuous exercise on free-recall memory. *Ergonomics, 30,* 121-129.

Travlos, A.K., & Marisi, D.Q. (1995). Information processing and concentration as a function of fitness level and exercise-induced activation to exhaustion. *Perceptual and Motor Skills, 80,* 15-26.

Van Boxtel, G.J., & Brunia, C.H. (1994). Motor and non-motor aspects of slow brain potentials. *Biological Psychology, 38,* 37-51.

Van Boxtel, G.J., Geraats, L.H., Van den Berg-Lenssen, M.M., & Brunia, C.H. (1993). Detection of EMG onset in ERP research. *Psychophysiology, 30,* 405-412.

Van Petten, C., & Luka, B.J. (2006). Neural localization of semantic context effects in electromagnetic and hemodynamic studies. *Brain and Language, 97,* 279-293.

Van Veen, V., & Carter, C.S. (2002). The timing of action-monitoring processes in the anterior cingulate cortex. *Journal of Cognitive Neuroscience, 14,* 593-602.

Vogel, E.K., & Luck, S.J. (2000). The visual N1 component as an index of a discrimination process. *Psychophysiology, 37,* 190-203.

Walsh, P., Kane, N., & Butler, S. (2005). The clinical role of evoked potentials. *Journal of Neurology, Neurosurgery, and Psychiatry, 76,* 16-22.

Walter, W.G., Cooper, R., Aldridge, V.J., McCallum, W.C., & Winter, A.L. (1964). Contingent negative variation: an electric sign of sensorimotor association and expectancy in the human brain. *Nature, 203,* 380-384.

Weerts, T.C., & Lang, P.J. (1973). The effects of eye fixation and stimulus and response location on the contingent negative variation (CNV). *Biological Psychology, 1,* 1-19.

Yagi, Y., Coburn, K.L., Estes, K.M., & Arruda, J.E. (1999). Effects of aerobic exercise and gender on visual and auditory P300, reaction time, and accuracy. *European Journal of Applied Physiology and Occupational Physiology, 80,* 402-408.

Yeung, N., Cohen, J.D., & Botvinick, M.M. (2004). The neural basis of error detection: conflict monitoring and the error-related negativity. *Psychological Review, 111,* 931-959.

Chapter 8

Archer, J.S., Love-Geffen, T.E., Herbst-Damm, K.L., Swinney, D.A., Chang, J.R. (2006). Effect of estradiol versus estradiol and testosterone on brain-activation patterns in postmenopausal women. *Menopause* 13(3): 528-537.

Bartenstein, P., Minoshima, S., Hirsch, C., Buch, K., Willoch, F., Mosch, D., Schad, D., Schwaiger, M., Kurz, A. (1997). Quantitative assessment of cerebral blood flow in patients with Alzheimer's disease by SPECT. *J Nucl Med* 38(7): 1095-1101.

Bentourkia, M., Bol, A., Ivanoiu, A., Labar, D., Sibomana, M., Coppens, A., Michel, C., Cosnard, G., De Volder, A.G. (2000). Comparison of regional blood flow and glucose metabolism in the normal brain: effect of aging. *J Neurol Sci* 181(1-2): 19-28.

Berchtold, N.C., Kesslak, J.P., Pike, C.J., Adlard, P.A., Cotman, C.W. (2001). Estrogen and exercise interact to regulate brain-derived neurotrophic factor mRNA and protein expression in the hippocampus. *Eur J Neurosci* 14(12): 1992-2002.

Biver, F., Lotstra, F., Monclus, M., Dethy, S., Damhaut, P., Wikler, D., Luxen, A., Goldman, S. (1997). In vivo binding of [18F]altanserin to rat brain 5HT2 receptors: a film and electronic autoradiographic study. *Nucl Med Biol* 24(4): 357-360.

Boccardi, M., Ghidoni, R., Govoni, S., Testa, C., Benussi, L., Bonetti, M., Binetti, G., Frisoni, G.B. (2006). Effects of hormone therapy on brain morphology of healthy postmenopausal women: a voxel-based morphometry study. *Menopause* 13(4): 584-591.

Bonte, F.J., Ross, E.D., Chehabi, H.H., Devous, M.D. (1986). SPECT study of regional cerebral blood flow in Alzheimer disease. *J Comput Assist Tomogr* 10(4): 579-583.

Brand, A., Richter-Landsberg, C., Leibfritz, D. (1993). Multinuclear NMR studies on the energy metabolism of glial and neuronal cells. *Dev Neurosci* 15: 289-298.

Brooks, J.C., Roberts, N., Kemp, G.J., Gosney, M.A., Lye, M., Whitehouse, G.H. (2001). A proton magnetic resonance spectroscopy study of age-related changes in frontal lobe metabolite concentrations. *Cereb Cortex* 11(7): 598-605.

Buckner, R.L., Snyder, A.Z., Shannon, B.J., LaRossa, G., Sachs, R., Fotenos, A.F., Sheline, Y.I., Klunk, W.E., Mathis, C.A., Morris, J.C., Mintun, M.A. (2005). Molecular, structural, and functional characterization of Alzheimer's disease: evidence for a relationship between default activity, amyloid, and memory. *J Neurosci* 25(34): 7709-7717.

Calvaresi, E., & Bryan, J. (2001). B vitamins, cognition, and aging: a review. *J Gerontol B Psychol Sci Soc Sci* 56(6): 327-339.

Chang, L., Ernst, T., Poland, R.E., Jenden, D.J. (1996). In vivo proton magnetic resonance spectroscopy of the normal aging human brain. *Life Sci* 58: 2049-2056.

References

Chantal, S., Braun, C.M., Bouchard, R.W., Labelle, M., Boulanger, Y. (2004). Similar 1H magnetic resonance spectroscopic metabolic pattern in the medial temporal lobes of patients with mild cognitive impairment and Alzheimer's disease. *Brain Res* 1003(1-2): 26-35.

Colcombe, S., & Kramer, A.F. (2003). Fitness effects on the cognitive function of older adults: a meta-analytic study. *Psychol Science* 14: 125-130.

Colcombe, S.J., Kramer, A.F., Erickson, K.I., Scalf, P. (2005). The implications of cortical recruitment and brain morphology for individual differences in inhibitory function in aging humans. *Psychol Aging* 20(3): 363-375.

Colcombe, S.J., Kramer, A.F., Erickson, K.I., Scalf, P., McAuley, E., Cohen, N.J., Webb, A., Jerome, G.J., Marquez, D.X., Elavsky, S. (2004). Cardiovascular fitness, cortical plasticity, and aging. *Proc Natl Acad Sci USA* 101(9): 3316-3321.

Cook, I.A., Morgan, M.L., Dunkin, J.J., David, S., Witte, E., Lufkin, R., Abrams, M., Rosenberg, S., Leuchter, A.F. (2002). Estrogen replacement therapy is associated with less progression of subclinical structural brain disease in normal elderly women: a pilot study. *Int J Geriat Psychiatry* 17(7): 610-618.

Cyr, M., Bosse, R., Di Paolo, T. (1998). Gonadal hormones modulate 5-hydroxytryptamine 2A receptors: emphasis on the rat frontal cortex. *Neuroscience* 83(3): 829-836.

Duka, T., Tasker, R., McGowan, J.F. (2000). The effects of 3-week estrogen hormone replacement on cognition in elderly healthy females. *Psychopharmacology* (Berl.) 149(2): 129-139.

Eberling, J.L., Jagust, W.J., Reed, B.R., Baker, M.G. (1992). Reduced temporal lobe blood flow in Alzheimer's disease. *Neurobiol Aging* 13(4): 483-491.

Eberling, J.L., Reed, B.R., Baker, M.G., Jagust, W.J. (1993). Cognitive correlates of regional cerebral blood flow in Alzheimer's disease. *Arch Neurol* 50(7): 761-766.

Eberling, J.L., Reed, B.R., Coleman, J.E., Jagust, W.J. (2000). Effect of estrogen on cerebral glucose metabolism in postmenopausal women. *Neurology* 55(6): 875-877.

Eberling, J.L., Wu, C., Haan, M.N., Mungas, D., Buonocore, M., Jagust, W.J. (2003). Preliminary evidence that estrogen protects against age-related hippocampal atrophy. *Neurobiol Aging* 24(5): 725-732.

Eberling, J.L., Wu, C., Tong-Turnbeaugh, R., Jagust, W.J. (2004). Estrogen- and tamoxifen-associated effects on brain structure and function. *NeuroImage* 21(1): 364-371.

Erickson, K.I., Colcombe, S.J., Elavsky, S., McAuley, E., Korol, D.L., Scalf, P.E., Kramer, A.F. (2007a). Interactive effects of fitness and hormone treatment on brain health in postmenopausal women. *Neurobiol Aging* 28(2): 179-185.

Erickson, K.I., Colcombe, S.J, Raz, N., Korol, D.L., Scalf, P., Webb, A., Cohen, N.J., McAuley, E., Kramer, A.F. (2005). Selective sparing of brain tissue in postmenopausal women receiving hormone replacement therapy. *Neurobiol Aging* 26(8): 1205-1213.

Erickson, K.I., Colcombe, S.J., Wadhwa, R., Bherer, L., Peterson, M.S., Scalf, P.E., Kim, J.S., Alvarado, M., Kramer, A.F. (2007b). Training-induced plasticity in older adults: effects of training on hemispheric activity. *Neurobiol Aging* 28(2): 272-283.

Erickson, K.I., Pruis, T.A., Debrey, S.M., Bohacek, J., Korol, D.L. (2006). Estrogen and exercise interact to up-regulate BDNF levels in the hippocampus but not striatum of middle-aged Brown-Norway rats. Program No. 266.17. *Soc Neurosci Abstr.*

Ernst, T., Chang, L., Cooray, D., Salvador, C., Jovicich, J., Walot, I., Boone, K., Chlebowski, R. (2002). The effects of tamoxifen and estrogen on brain metabolism in elderly women. *J Natl Cancer Inst* 94(8): 592-597.

Friedland, R.P., Budinger, T.F., Ganz, E., Yano, Y., Mathis, C.A., Koss, B., Ober, B.A., Huesman, R.H., Derenzo, S.E. (1983). Regional cerebral metabolic alterations in dementia of the Alzheimer type: positron emission tomography with [18F] fluorodeoxyglucose. *J Compu Assist Tomogr* 7(4): 590-598.

Fukui, K., Omoi, N.O., Hayasaka, T., Shinnkai, T., Suzuki, S., Abe, K., Urano, S. (2002). Cognitive impairment of rats caused by oxidative stress and aging, and its prevention by vitamin E. *Ann NY Acad Sci* 959: 275-284.

Funk, J., Mortel, K., Meyer, J. (1991). Effects of estrogen replacement therapy on cerebral perfusion and cognition among postmenopausal women. *Dementia* 2: 268-272.

Gibbs, R.B., & Gabor, R. (2003). Estrogen and cognition: applying preclinical findings to clinical perspectives. *J Neurosci Res* 74(5): 637-643.

Gibbs, R.B., Hashash, A., Johnson, D.A. (1997). Effects of estrogen on potassium-stimulated acetylcholine release in the hippocampus and overlying cortex of adult rats. *Brain Res* 749(1): 143-146.

Goekoop, R., Rombouts, S.A., Jonker, C., Hibbel, A., Knol, D.L., Truyen, L., Barkhof, F., Scheltens, P. (2004). Challenging the cholinergic system in mild cognitive impairment: a pharmacological fMRI study. *NeuroImage* 23(4): 1450-1459.

Gould, E., Woolley, C.S., Frankfurt, M., McEwen, B.S. (1990). Gonadal steroids regulate dendritic spine density in hippocampal pyramidal cells in adulthood. *J Neurosci* 10(4): 1286-1291.

Greenberg, D.L., Payne, M.E., MacFall, J.R., Provenzale, J.M., Steffens, D.C., Krishnan, R.R. (2006). Differences in brain volumes among males and female hormone-therapy users and nonusers. *Psychiatry Res* 147(2-3): 127-134.

Greene, R.A. (2000). Estrogen and cerebral blood flow: a mechanism to explain the impact of estrogen on the incidence and treatment of Alzheimer's disease. *Int J Fertil Women's Med* 45(4): 253-257.

Ha, D.M., Xu, J., Janowsky, J.S. (2007). Preliminary evidence that long-term estrogen use reduces white matter loss in aging. *Neurobiol Aging.* 28: 1936-1940.

References

Henderson, V.W. (2006). Estrogen-containing hormone therapy and Alzheimer's disease risk: understanding discrepant inferences from observational and experimental research. *Neuroscience* 138(3): 1031-1039.

Hogervorst, E., Williams, J., Budge, M., Riedel, W., Jolles, J. (2000). The nature of the effect of female gonadal hormone replacement therapy on cognitive function in post-menopausal women: a meta-analysis. *Neuroscience* 101(3): 485-512.

Hogh, P., Knudsen, G.M., Kjaer, K.H., Jorgensen, O.S., Paulson, O.B., Waldemar, G. (2001). Single photon emission computed tomography and apolipoprotein E in Alzheimer's disease: impact of the epsilon4 allele on regional cerebral blood flow. *J Geriatr Psychiatry Neurol* 14(1): 42-51.

Hu, L., Yue, Y., Zuo, P.P., Jin, Z.Y., Feng, F., You, H., Li, M.L., Ge, Q.S. (2006). Evaluation of neuroprotective effects of long-term low dose hormone replacement therapy on postmenopausal women brain hippocampus using magnetic resonance scanner. *Chin Med Sci J* 21(4): 214-218.

Joffe, H., Hall, J.E., Gruber, S., Sarmiento, I.A., Cohen, L.S., Yurgelun-Todd, D., Martin, K.A. (2006). Estrogen therapy selectively enhances prefrontal cognitive processes: a randomized, double-blind, placebo-controlled study with functional magnetic resonance imaging in perimenopausal and recently postmenopausal women. *Menopause* 13(3): 411-422.

Kantarci, K., Smith, G.E., Ivnik, R.J., Peterson, R.C., Boeve, B.F., Knopman, D.S., Tangalos, E.G., Jack, C.R. (2002). 1H magnetic resonance spectroscopy, cognitive function, and apolipoprotein E genotype in normal aging, mild cognitive impairment and Alzheimer's disease. *J Int Neuropsychol Soc* 8(7): 934-942.

Korol, D.L. (2004). Role of estrogen in balancing contributions from multiple memory systems. *Neurobiol Learn Mem* 82(3): 309-323.

Korol, D.L., & Pruis, T.A. (2004). Estrogen and exercise modulate learning strategy in middle-aged female rats. Program No. 770.7. *Soc Neurosci Abstr.*

Kramer, A.F., & Erickson, K.I. (in press). Capitalizing on cortical plasticity: influence of physical activity on cognition and brain function. *Trends Cogn Sci.* E-pub ahead of print.

Krause, D.N., Duckles, S.P., Pelligrino, D.A. (2006). Influence of sex steroid hormones on cerebrovascular function. *J Appl Physiol* 101(4): 1252-1261.

Kugaya, A., Epperson, C.N., Zoghbi, S., van Dyck, C.H., Hou, Y., Fugita, M., Staley, J.K., Garg, P.K., Seibyl, J.P., Innis, R.B. (2003). Increase in prefrontal cortex serotonin 2A receptors following estrogen treatment in postmenopausal women. *Am J Psychiatry* 160(8): 1522-1524.

Kuhl, D.E., Minoshima, S., Fessler, J.A., Frey, K.A., Foster, N.L., Ficaro, E.P., Wieland, D.M., Koeppe, R.A. (1996). In vivo mapping of cholinergic terminals in normal aging, Alzheimer's disease, and Parkinson's disease. *Ann Neurol* 40(3): 399-410.

Lemaire, C., Cantineau, R., Guillaume, M., Plenevaux, A., Christiaens, L. (1991). Fluorine-18-altanserin: a radioligand for the study of serotonin receptors with

PET: radiolabeling and in vivo biologic behavior in rats. *J Nucl Med* 32(12): 2266-2272.

Lord, C., Buss, C., Lupien, S.J., Pruessner, J.C. (2006). Hippocampal volumes are larger in postmenopausal women using estrogen therapy compared to past users, never users and men: a possible window of opportunity effect. *Neurobiol Aging*. E-pub ahead of print.

Low, L.F., Anstey, K.J., Maller, J., Kumar, R., Wen, W., Lux, O., Salonikas, C., Naidoo, D., Sachdev, P. (2006). Hormone replacement therapy, brain volumes and white matter in postmenopausal women aged 60-64 years. *Neuroreport* 17(1): 101-104.

Lu, B., Pang, P.T., Woo, N.H. (2005). The yin and yang of neurotrophin action. *Nature Neuroscience* 6: 603-614.

Luine, V., Park, D., Joh, T., Reis, D., McEwen, B. (1980). Immunochemical demonstration of increased choline acetyltransferase concentration in rat preoptic area after estradiol administration. *Brain Res* 191(1): 273-277.

Luoto, R., Manolio, T., Meilahn, E., Bhadelia, R., Furberg, C., Cooper, L., Kraut, M. (2000). Estrogen replacement therapy and MRI-demonstrated cerebral infarcts, white matter changes, and brain atrophy in older women: the Cardiovascular Health Study. *J Am Geriatr Soc* 48(5): 467-472.

Maki, P.M. (2006). Hormone therapy and cognitive function: is there a critical period for benefit? *Neuroscience* 138(3): 1027-1030.

Maki, P.M., & Resnick, S.M. (2000). Longitudinal effects of estrogen replacement therapy on PET cerebral blood flow and cognition. *Neurobiol Aging* 21: 373-383.

Martin, A.J., Friston, K.J., Colebatch, J.G., Frackowiak, R.S. (1991). Decreases in regional cerebral blood flow with normal aging. *J Cereb Blood Flow Metab* 11(4): 684-689.

Maki, P.M., Zonderman, A.B., Resnick, S.M. (2001). Enhanced verbal memory in nondemented elderly women receiving hormone-replacement therapy. *Am J Psychiatry* 158(2): 227-233.

Marriott, L.K., Hauss-Wegrzyniak, B., Benton, R.S., Vraniak, P., Wenk, G.L. (2002). Long term estrogen therapy worsens the behavioral and neuropathological consequences of chronic brain in flammation. *Behavioral Neuroscience* 116: 902-911.

Marriott, L.K., & Korol, D.L. (2003). Short-term estrogen treatment in ovariectomized rats augments hippocampal acetylcholine release during place learning. *Neurobiol Learn Mem* 80: 315-322.

Mega, M.S., Cummings, J.L., O'Conner, S.M., Dinov, I.D., Reback, E., Felix, J., Masterman, D.L., Phelps, M.E., Small, G.W., Toga, A.W. (2001). Cognitive and metabolic responses to metrifonate therapy in Alzheimer disease. *Neuropsychiatry Neuropsychol Behav Neurol* 14(1): 63-68.

Melamed, E., Lavy, S., Bentin, S., Cooper, G., Rinot, Y. (1980). Reduction in regional cerebral blood flow during normal aging in man. *Stroke* 11(1): 31-35.

References

Meltzer, C.C., Smith, G., Price, J.C., Reynolds, C.F., Mathis, C.A., Greer, P., Lopresti, B., Mintun, M.A., Pollock, B.G., Ben-Eliezer, D., Cantwell, M.N., Kaye, W., DeKosky, S.T. (1998). Reduced binding of [18F]altanserin to serotonin type 2A receptors in aging: persistence of effect after partial volume correction. *Brain Res* 813(1): 167-171.

Miller, M.M., Monjan, A.A., Buckholtz, N.S. (2001). Estrogen replacement therapy for the potential treatment or prevention of Alzheimer's disease. *Ann NY Acad Sci* 949: 223-234.

Mintun, M.A., Sheline, Y.I., Moerlein, S.M., Vlassenko, A.G., Huang, Y., Snyder, A.Z. (2004). Decreased hippocampal 5-HT2A receptor binding in major depressive disorder: in vivo measurement with [18F]altanserin positron emission tomography. *Biol Psychiatry* 55(3): 217-224.

Montaldi, D., Brooks, D.N., McColl, J.H., Wyper, D., Patterson, J., Barron, E., McCulloch, J. (1990). Measurements of regional cerebral blood flow and cognitive performance in Alzheimer's disease. *J Neurol Neurosurg Psychiatry* 53(1): 33-38.

Moses, E.L., Drevets, W.C., Smith, G., Mathis, C.A., Kalro, B.N., Butters, M.A., Leondires, M.P., Greer, P.J., Lopresti, B., Loucks, T.L., Berga, S.L. (2000). Effects of estradiol and progesterone administration on human serotonin 2A receptor binding: a PET study. *Biol Psychiatry* 48(8): 854-860.

Moses-Kolko, E.L., Berga, S.L., Greer, P.J., Smith, G., Meltzer, C.C., Drevets, W.C. (2003). Widespread increases of cortical serotonin type 2A receptor availability after hormone therapy in euthymic postmenopausal women. *Fertil Steril* 80(3): 554-559.

Nobili, F., Copello, F., Buffoni, F., Vitali, P., Girtler, N., Bordoni, C., Safaie-Semnani, E., Mariani, G., Rodriguez, G. (2001). Regional cerebral blood flow and prognostic evaluation in Alzheimer's disease. *Dement Geriatr Cogn Disord* 12(2): 89-97.

Nobili, F., Vitali, P., Canfora, M., Girtler, N., De Leo, C., Mariani, G., Pupi, A., Rodriguez, G. (2002). Effects of long-term Donepezil therapy on rCBF of Alzheimer's patients. *Clin Neurophysiol* 113(8): 1241-1248.

Nordberg, A., Lilja, A., Lundqvist, H., Hartvig, P., Amberla, K., Viitanen, M., Warpman, U., Johansson, M., Hellstrom-Lindahl, E., Bjurling, P., et al. (1992). Tacrine restores cholinergic nicotinic receptors and glucose metabolism in Alzheimer patients as visualized by positron emission tomography. *Neurobiol Aging* 13(6): 747-758.

Ohkura, T., Isse, K., Akazawa, K., Hamamoto, M., Yaoi, Y., Hagino, N. (1994). Evaluation of estrogen treatment in female patients with dementia of the Alzheimer type. *Endocr J* 41(4): 361-371.

Ohkura, T., Teshima, Y., Isse, K., Matsuda, H., Inoue, T., Sakai, Y., Iwasaki, N., Yaoi, Y. (1995). Estrogen increases cerebral and cerebellar blood flows in postmenopausal women. *Menopause* 2: 13-18.

Potkin, S.G., Anand, R., Fleming, K., Alva, G., Keator, D., Carreon, D., Messina, J., Wu, J.C., Hartman, R., Fallon, J.H. (2001). Brain metabolic and clinical effects of rivastigmine in Alzheimer's disease. *Int J Neuropsychopharmacol* 4(3): 223-230.

Prohovnik, I., Mayeux, R., Sackeim, H.A., Smith, G., Stern, Y., Alderson, P.O. (1988). Cerebral perfusion as a diagnostic marker of early Alzheimer's disease. *Neurology* 38(6): 931-937.

Rapp, S., Espeland, M., Shumaker, S., Henderson, V., Brunner, R., Manson, J., Gass, M., Stefanick, M., Lane, D., Hays, J., Johnson, K., Coker, L., Dailey, M., Bowen, D. (2003). Effect of estrogen plus progestin on global cognitive function in postmenopausal women: the Women's Health Initiative Memory Study: a randomized controlled trial. *JAMA* 289: 2663-2672.

Rasgon, N.L., Silverman, D., Siddarth, P., Miller, K., Ercoli, L.M., Elman, S., Lavretsky, H., Huang, S.C., Phelps, M.E., Small, G.W. (2005). Estrogen use and brain metabolic change in postmenopausal women. *Neurobiol Aging* 26(2): 229-235.

Rasgon, N.L., Small, G.W., Siddarth, P., Miller, K., Ercoli, L.M., Bookheimer, S.Y., Lavretsky, H., Huang, S.C., Barrio, J.R., Phelps, M.E. (2001). Estrogen use and brain metabolic change in older adults. A preliminary report. *Psychiatry Res* 107(1): 11-18.

Raz, N., Gunning-Dixon, F., Head, D., Rodrigue, K.M., Williamson, A., Acker, J.D. (2004a). Aging, sexual dimorphism, and hemispheric asymmetry of the cerebral cortex: replicability of regional differences in volume. *Neurobiol Aging* 25(3): 377-396.

Raz, N., & Rodrigue, K.M. (2006). Differential aging of the brain: patterns, cognitive correlates and modifiers. *Neurosci Biobehav Rev* 30(6): 730-748.

Raz, N., Rodrigue, K.M., Kennedy, K.M., Acker, J.D. (2004b). Hormone replacement therapy and age-related brain shrinkage: regional effects. *Neuroreport* 15(16): 2531-2534.

Resnick, S.M., Coker, L.H., Maki, P.M., Rapp, S.R., Espeland, M.A., Shumaker, S.A. (2006a). The Women's Health Initiative Study of Cognitive Aging (WHISCA): a randomized clinical trial of the effects of hormone therapy on age-related cognitive decline. *Clin Trials* 1: 440-450.

Resnick, S.M., Maki, P.M., Golski, S., Kraut, M.A., Zonderman, A.B. (1998). Estrogen effects on PET cerebral blood flow and neuropsychological performance. *Horm Behav* 34: 171-184.

Resnick, S.M., Maki, P.M., Rapp, S.R., Espeland, M.A., Brunner, R., Coker, L.H., Granek, I.A., Hogan, P., Ockene, J.K., Shumaker, S.A. (2006b). Effects of combination estrogen plus progestin hormone treatment on cognition and affect. *J Clin Endocrinol Metab* 91: 1802-1810.

Robertson, D.M., van Amelsvoort, T., Daly, E., Simmons, A., Whitehead, M., Morris, R.G., Murphy, K.C., Murphy, D.G. (2001). Effects of estrogen replacement therapy on human brain aging: an in vivo 1H MRS study. *Neurology* 57(11): 2114-2117.

Rossouw, J.E., Prentice, R.L., Manson, J.E., Wu, L., Barad, D., Barnabei, V.M., Ko, M., LaCroix, A.Z., Margolis, K.L., Stefanick, M.L. (2007). Postmenopausal hormone therapy and risk of cardiovascular disease by age and years since menopause. *JAMA* 297(13): 1465-77.

References

Sakamoto, S., Matsuda, H., Asada, T., Ohnishi, T., Nakano, S., Kanetaka, H., Takasaki, M. (2003). Apoliprotein E genotype and early Alzheimer's disease: a longitudinal SPECT study. *J Neuroimaging* 13(2): 113-123.

Schmidt, R., Fazekas, F., Reinhart, B., Kapeller, P., Fazekas, G., Offenbacher, H., Eber, B., Schumacher, M., Freidl, W. (1996). Estrogen replacement therapy in older women: a neuropsychological and brain MRI study. *J Am Geriat Soc* 44(11): 1307-1313.

Schooler, C., & Mulatu, M.S. (2001). The reciprocal effects of leisure time activities and intellectual functioning in older people: a longitudinal analysis. *Psychol Aging* 16(3): 466-482.

Shaywitz, S.E., Shaywitz, B.A., Pugh, K.R., Fulbright, R.K., et al. (1999). Effect of estrogen on brain activation patterns in postmenopausal women during working memory tasks. *JAMA* 281(13): 1197-1202.

Sherwin, B.B. (2003). Estrogen and cognitive functioning in women. *Endocr Rev* 24(2): 133-151.

Sherwin, B.B. (2006). Estrogen and cognitive aging in women. *Neuroscience* 138(3): 1021-1026.

Shumaker, S.A., Legault, C., Kuller, L., Rapp, S., Thal, L., Lane, D., Fillit, H., Stefanick, M., Hendrix, S., Lewis, C.B., Masaki, K., Coker, L. (2004). Conjugated equine estrogens and incidence of probable dementia and mild cognitive impairment in postmenopausal women. *JAMA* 291: 2947-2958.

Shumaker, S.A., Legault, C., Thal, L., Wallace, R., Ockene, J., Hendrix, S., Jones, III, B., Assaf, A., Jackson, R., Kotchen, J.M., Wassertheil-Smoller, S., Wactawski-Wende, J. (2003). Estrogen plus progestin and the incidence of dementia and mild cognitive impairment in postmenopausal women: the Women's Health Initiative Memory Study: a randomized controlled trial. *JAMA* 289: 2651-2662.

Slopien, R., Junik, R., Meczekalski, B., Halerz-Nowakowska, B., Maciejewska, M., Warenik-Szymankiewicz, A., Sowinski, J. (2003). Influence of hormonal replacement therapy on the regional cerebral blood flow in postmenopausal women. *Maturitas* 46(4): 255-262.

Small, G.W., Ercoli, L.M., Silverman, D.H., Huang, S.C., Komo, S., Bookheimer, S.Y., Lavretsky, H., Miller, K., et al. (2000). Cerebral metabolic and cognitive decline in persons at genetic risk for Alzheimer's disease. *Proc Natl Acad Sci USA* 97(11): 6037-6042.

Small, G.W., Mazziotta, J.C., Collins, M.T., Baxter, L.R., Phelps, M.E., Mandelkern, M.A., Kaplan, A., La Rue, A., Adamson, C.F., Chang, L., et al. (1995). Apolipoprotein E type 4 allele and cerebral glucose metabolism in relatives at risk for familial Alzheimer disease. *JAMA* 273 (12): 942-947.

Smith, G.S., Price, J.C., Lopresti, B.J., Huang, Y., Simpson, N., Holt, D., Mason, N.S., Meltzer, C.C., Sweet, R.A., Nichols, T., Sashin, D., Mathis, C.A. (1998). Test-retest variability of serotonin 5-HT2A receptor binding measured with positron emission tomography and [18F]altanserin in the human brain. *Synapse* 30(4): 380-392.

Smith, Y.R., Love, T., Persad, C.C., Tkaczyk, A., Nichols, T.E., Zubieta, J.K. (2006). Impact of combined estradiol and norethindrone therapy on visuospatial working memory assessed by functional magnetic resonance imaging. *J Clin Endocrinol Metab* 91(11): 4476-4481.

Smith, Y.R., Minoshima, S., Kuhl, D.E., Zubieta, J.K. (2001). Effects of long-term hormone therapy on cholinergic synaptic concentrations in healthy postmenopausal women. *J Clin Endocrinol Metab* 86(2): 679-684.

Staff, R.T., Gemmell, H.G., Shanks, M.F., Murray, A.D., Venneri, A. (2000). Changes in the rCBF images of patients with Alzheimer's disease receiving Donepezil therapy. *Nucl Med Commun* 21(1): 37-41.

Stevens, M.C., Clark, V.P., Prestwood, K.M. (2005). Low-dose estradiol alters brain activity. *Psychiatry Res* 139(3): 199-217.

Sullivan, E.V., Marsh, L., Pfefferbaum, A. (2005). Preservation of hippocampal volume throughout adulthood in healthy men and women. *Neurobiol Aging* 26(7): 1093-1098.

Sumner, B.E., & Fink, G. (1997). The density of 5-hydroxytryptamine 2A receptors in forebrain is increased at pro-oestrus in intact female rats. *Neuroscience Letters* 234(1): 7-10.

Tanaka, S., Kawamata, J., Shimohama, S., Akahi, H., Akiguchi, I., Kimura, J., Ueda, K. (1998). Inferior temporal lobe atrophy and APOE genotypes in Alzheimer's disease. X-ray computed tomography, magnetic resonance imaging and Xe-133 SPECT studies. *Dement Geriatr Cogn Disord* 9(2): 90-98.

Tanapat, P., Hastings, N.B., Reeves, A.J., Gould, E. (1999). Estrogen stimulates a transient increase in the number of new neurons in the dentate gyrus of the adult female rat. *J Neurosci* 19(14): 5792-5801.

Wang, P.N., Liao, S.Q., Liu, R.S., Liu, C.Y., Chao, H.T., Lu, S.R., Yu, H.Y., Wang, S.J., Liu, H.C. (2000). Effects of estrogen on cognition, mood, and cerebral blood flow in AD: a controlled study. *Neurology* 54: 2061-2066.

Wilson, R.S., Mendes de Leon, C.F., Barnes, L.L., Schneider, J.A., Bienias, J.L., Evans, D.A., et al. (2002). Participation in cognitive stimulating activities and risk of incident Alzheimer's disease. *JAMA* 287: 742-748.

Zec, R.F., & Trivedi, M.A. (2002). The effects of estrogen replacement therapy on neuropsychological functioning in postmenopausal women with and without dementia: a critical and theoretical review. *Neuropsychol Rev* 12(2): 65-109.

Chapter 9

Abbott, R.D., White, L.R., Ross, G.W., Masaki, K.H., Curb, J.D., & Petrovitch, H. (2004). Walking and dementia in physically capable elderly men. *Journal of the American Medical Association, 292*(12), 1447-1453.

Albert, M.S., Jones, K., Savage, C.R., Berkman, L., Seeman, T., Blazer, D., et al. (1995). Predictors of cognitive change in older persons: MacArthur Studies of Successful Aging. *Psychology and Aging, 10*(4), 578-589.

References

Barnes, D.E., Yaffe, K., Satariano, W.A., & Tager, I.B. (2003). A longitudinal study of cardiorespiratory fitness and cognitive function in healthy older adults. *Journal of the American Geriatrics Society, 51*(4), 459-465.

Blaney, J., Sothmann, M., Raff, H., Hart, B., & Horn, T. (1990). Impact of exercise training on plasma adrenocorticotropin response to a well-learned vigilance task. *Psychoneuroendocrinology, 15*(5-6), 453-462.

Blomquist, K.B., & Danner, F. (1987). Effects of physical conditioning on information-processing efficiency. *Perceptual and Motor Skills, 65*, 175-186.

Blumenthal, J.A., & Madden, D.J. (1988). Effects of aerobic exercise training, age, and physical-fitness on memory-search performance. *Psychology and Aging, 3*(3), 280-285.

Colcombe, S., & Kramer, A.F. (2003). Fitness effects on the cognitive function of older adults: a meta-analytic study. *Psychological Science, 14*(2), 125-130.

Colcombe, S.J., Kramer, A.F., Erickson, K.I., Scalf, P., McAuley, E., Cohen, N.J., et al. (2004). Cardiovascular fitness, cortical plasticity, and aging. *Proceedings of the National Academy of Sciences USA, 101*(9), 3316-3321.

Dik, M.G., Deeg, D.J.H., Visser, M., & Jonker, C. (2003). Early life physical activity and cognition at old age. *Journal of Clinical and Experimental Neuropsychology, 25*(5), 643-653.

Dustman, R.E., Ruhling, R.O., Russell, E.M., Shearer, D.E., Bonekat, H.W., Shigeoka, J.W., et al. (1984). Aerobic exercise training and improved neuropsychological function of older individuals. *Neurobiology of Aging, 5*(1), 35-42.

El-Naggar, A.M. (1986). Physical training effect on relationship of physical, mental, and emotional fitness in adult men. *Journal of Human Ergology, 15*, 79-84.

Emery, C.F., Schein, R.L., Hauck, E.R., & MacIntyre, N.R. (1998). Psychological and cognitive outcomes of a randomized trial of exercise among patients with chronic obstructive pulmonary disease. *Health Psychology, 17*(3), 232-240.

Emery, C.F., Shermer, R.L., Hauck, E.R., Hsiao, E.T., & MacIntyre, N.R. (2003). Cognitive and psychological outcomes of exercise in a 1-year follow-up study of patients with chronic obstructive pulmonary disease. *Health Psychology, 22*(6), 598-604.

Etnier, J.L. (2008). Mediators of the exercise and cognition relationship. In: W.W. Spirduso, W. Chodzko-Zajko, & L.W. Poon. (Eds), *Aging, exercise, and cognition series: Vol. 2. Exercise and its mediating effects on cognition* (pp. 13-32). Champaign, IL: Human Kinetics.

Etnier, J.L., & Berry, M. (2001). Fluid intelligence in an older COPD sample after short- or long-term exercise. *Medicine and Science in Sports and Exercise, 33*(10), 1620-1628.

Etnier, J.L., Salazar, W., Landers, D.M., Petruzzello, S.J., Han, M., & Nowell, P. (1997). The influence of physical fitness and exercise upon cognitive functioning: a meta-analysis. *Journal of Sport and Exercise Psychology, 19*, 249-277.

References

Harma, M.I., Ilmarinen, J., Knauth, P., Rutenfranz, J., & Hanninen, O. (1988). Physical-training intervention in female shift workers. 2. The effects of intervention on the circadian-rhythms of alertness, short-term-memory, and body-temperature. *Ergonomics, 31*(1), 51-63.

Hascelik, Z., Basgoze, O., Turker, K., Narman, S., & Ozker, R. (1989). The effects of physical training on physical fitness tests and auditory and visual reaction times of volleyball players. *Journal of Sports Medicine and Physical Fitness, 29*, 234-239.

Hassmen, P., Ceci, R., & Backman, L. (1992). Exercise for older women: a training method and its influences on physical and cognitive performance. *European Journal of Applied Physiology and Occupational Physiology, 64*(5), 460-466.

Heyn, P., Abreu, B.C., & Ottenbacher, K.J. (2004). The effects of exercise training on elderly persons with cognitive impairment and dementia: a meta-analysis. *Archives of Physical and Medical Rehabilitation, 85*(10), 1694-1704.

Hill, R.D., Storandt, M., & Malley, M. (1993). The impact of long-term exercise training on psychological function in older adults. *Journal of Gerontology, 48*(1), P12-P17.

Ismail, A.H., & El-Naggar, A.M. (1981). Effect of exercise on cognitive processing in adult men. *Journal of Human Ergology, 10*, 83-91.

Khatri, P., Blumenthal, J.A., Babyak, M.A., Craighead, W.E., Herman, S., Baldewicz, T., et al. (2001). Effects of exercise training on cognitive functioning among depressed older men and women. *Journal of Aging and Physical Activity, 9*, 43-57.

Kramer, A.F., Hahn, S., McAuley, E., Cohen, N.J., Banich, M.T., Harrison, C., et al. (2002). Exercise, aging, and cognition: healthy body, healthy mind? In W.A. Rogers & A.D. Fisk (Eds.), *Human factors interventions for the health care of older adults* (pp. 91-120). Mahwah, NJ: Erlbaum.

Laurin, D., Verreault, R., Lindsay, J., MacPherson, K., & Rockwood, K. (2001). Physical activity and risk of cognitive impairment and dementia in elderly persons. *Archives of Neurology, 58*(3), 498-504.

Madden, D.J., Allen, P.A., Blumenthal, J.A., & Emery, C.F. (1989). Improving aerobic capacity in healthy older adults does not necessarily lead to improved cognitive performance. *Psychology and Aging, 4*(3), 307-320.

Moul, J.L., Goldman, B., & Warren, B. (1995). Physical activity and cognitive performance in the older population. *Journal of Aging and Physical Activity, 3*, 135-145.

Panton, L.B., Graves, J.E., Pollock, M.L., Hagberg, J.M., & Chen, W. (1990). Effect of aerobic and resistance training on fractionated reaction time and speed of movement. *Journal of Gerontology, 45*(1), M26-M31.

Pierce, T.W., Madden, D.J., Siegel, W.C., & Blumenthal, J.A. (1993). Effects of aerobic exercise on cognitive and psychosocial functioning in patients with mild hypertension. *Health Psychology, 12*(4), 286-291.

Podewils, L.J., Guallar, E., Kuller, L.H., Fried, L.P., Lopez, O.L., Carlson, M., et al. (2005). Physical activity, APOE genotype, and dementia risk: findings from the Cardiovascular Health Cognition Study. *American Journal of Epidemiology, 161*(7), 639-651.

References

Sibley, B.A., & Etnier, J.L. (2003). The relationship between physical activity and cognition in children: a meta-analysis. *Pediatric Exercise Science, 15*(3), 243-256.

van Gelder, B.M., Tijhuis, M.A., Kalmijn, S., Giampaoli, S., Nissinen, A., & Kromhout, D. (2004). Physical activity in relation to cognitive decline in elderly men: the FINE Study. *Neurology, 63*(12), 2316-2321.

Verghese, J., Lipton, R.B., Katz, M.J., Hall, C.B., Derby, C.A., Kuslansky, G., et al. (2003). Leisure activities and the risk of dementia in the elderly. *New England Journal of Medicine, 348*(25), 2508-2516.

Weuve, J., Kang, J.H., Manson, J.E., Breteler, M.M., Ware, J.H., & Grodstein, F. (2004). Physical activity, including walking, and cognitive function in older women. *Journal of the American Medical Association, 292*(12), 1454-1461.

Whitehurst, M. (1991). Reaction time unchanged in older women following aerobic training. *Perceptual and Motor Skills, 72,* 251-256.

Wilson, R.S., Bennett, D.A., Bienias, J.L., Aggarwal, N.T., Mendes De Leon, C.F., Morris, M.C., et al. (2002). Cognitive activity and incident AD in a population-based sample of older persons. *Neurology, 59*(12), 1910-1914.

Yaffe, K., Barnes, D., Nevitt, M., Lui, L.Y., & Covinsky, K. (2001). A prospective study of physical activity and cognitive decline in elderly women who walk. *Archives of Internal Medicine, 161*(14), 1703-1708.

Zervas, Y., Danis, A., & Klissouras, V. (1991). Influence of physical exertion on mental performance with reference to training. *Perceptual and Motor Skills, 72*(3), 1215-1221.

INDEX

Note: The italicized *f* and *t* following page numbers refer to figures and tables, respectively.

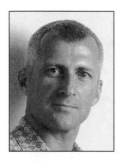

Wojtek Chodzko-Zajko, PhD, serves as both department head and professor of kinesiology and community health at the University of Illinois at Urbana-Champaign. He served on the World Health Organization Scientific Advisory Committee, which issued guidelines for physical activity for older adults. Chodzko-Zajko chairs the Active Aging Partnership, a national coalition in the area of healthy aging linking the American College of Sports Medicine, the National Institute of Aging, the Centers for Disease Control and Prevention, the American Geriatrics Society, the National Council on Aging, the American Association of Retired Persons, and the Robert Wood Johnson Foundation.

Since 2002, Chodzko-Zajko has served as principal investigator of the National Blueprint Project, a coalition of more than 50 national organizations with a joint commitment to promoting independent, active aging in the 50-plus population. He was founding editor of the *Journal of Aging and Physical Activity* and president of the International Society for Aging and Physical Activity.

He is frequently invited to speak about healthful aging at national and international meetings. Chodzko-Zajko has appeared often on television and radio, including the NBC *Today Show*, National Public Radio, and CNN.

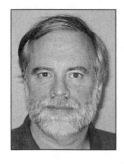

Arthur F. Kramer, PhD, holds the Swanlund endowed chair at the University of Illinois. Kramer is a fellow in the American Psychological Association and the American Psychological Society and is a member of the executive committee of the International Attention and Performance Society. He is also the director of the Biomedical Imaging Center, codirector of the NIH Roybal Center for Healthy Minds, and a professor of psychology and neuroscience at the Beckman Institute at the University of Illinois.

A major focus of research at Dr. Kramer's lab is the understanding and enhancement of cognitive and neural plasticity across the life span. Dr. Kramer served as an associate editor of *Perception and Psychophysics* and is currently a member of seven editorial boards. He is a recent recipient of the NIH Ten-Year MERIT Award. Kramer's research has been featured in numerous print, radio, and electronic media: the *New York Times, Wall Street*

Journal, Washington Post, Chicago Tribune, CBS Evening News, Today Show, NPR, and *Saturday Night Live.*

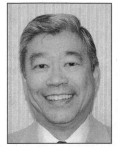

Leonard W. Poon, PhD, is a professor of public health and psychology, chair of the faculty of gerontology, and director of the Gerontology Center at the University of Georgia at Athens. He received his PhD in experimental psychology in 1972 from the University of Denver and has studied aging and cognition for over 30 years with specific emphasis on environmental and lifestyle influences that enhance cognitive functioning in older adults.

A fellow of the American Psychological Association, American Psychological Society, Association of Gerontology in Higher Education, and the Gerontology Society of America, Poon was a Fulbright senior research scholar in Sweden and a senior visiting research scientist to Japan. In 2000, Poon received an honorary doctorate of philosophy from Lund University in Sweden. Among his research awards are the NIA Special Research Award, VA Medical Research Service Achievement Award, North American Leader in Psychogeriatrics, and Southern Gerontological Society Academic Gerontologist Award.

Poon's primary research areas are normal and pathological changes of memory processes in aging, clinical assessment of memory (including assessment of early stages of dementia of the Alzheimer's type), and survival characteristics and adaptation of centenarians. He is currently directing a nine-university, NIA-funded program studying the genetic basis of longevity, relationships between the brain and behavior in Alzheimer's disease, and daily functioning capacities of the oldest old.

Poon currently resides in Athens, Georgia. In his free time he enjoys cycling, photography, and traveling.

Human Kinetics' Aging, Exercise, and Cognition Series

This series presents advanced research and key issues for understanding and researching the links between exercise, aging, and cognition. These three volumes are essential references for cognitive gerontologists; medical, health, and exercise science researchers and professionals; and public health administrators interested in scientific evidence demonstrating the beneficial effects of regular physical activity on cognitive functioning and general health during aging.

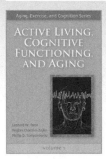

In *Active Living, Cognitive Functioning, and Aging*, internationally known experts present the status and future directions of research related to aging, physical activity, cognition, and putative mechanisms. The text discusses the potential of intervention programs that positively influence cognition and implications for public policy making for healthier older adults.

Active Living, Cognitive Functioning, and Aging
Leonard W. Poon, PhD, Wojtek Chodzko-Zajko, PhD, and Phillip D. Tomporowski, PhD, Editors
©2006 • Hardback • 264 pp • ISBN 978-0-7360-5785-1

Exercise and Its Mediating Effects on Cognition examines how physical activity can indirectly affect cognitive function by influencing mediators—such as sleep quality, nutrition, disease states, anxiety, and depression—that affect physical and mental resources for cognition.

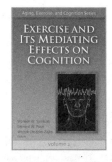

Exercise and Its Mediating Effects on Cognition
Waneen W. Spirduso, PhD, Leonard W. Poon, PhD, and Wojtek Chodzko-Zajko, PhD, Editors
©2008 • Hardback • 296 pp • ISBN 978-0-7360-5786-8

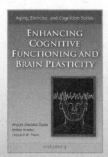

Enhancing Cognitive Functioning and Brain Plasticity examines exercise and nonexercise interventions shown to influence cognition and brain plasticity. The text discusses how state-of-the-art neuroimaging measures, including event-related brain potentials, positron emission tomography, and functional magnetic resonance imaging, are used in the study of individual differences in cognition and brain functioning.

Enhancing Cognitive Functioning and Brain Plasticity
Wojtek Chodzko-Zajko, PhD, Arthur Kramer, PhD, and Leonard W. Poon, PhD, Editors
©2009 • Hardback • Approx. 240 pp • ISBN 978-0-7360-5791-2

For more information, call (800) 747-4457 US • (800) 465-7301 CDN
44 (0) 113-255-5665 UK • (08) 8372-0999 AUS • (09) 448-1207 NZ • (217) 351-5076 International
Or visit **www.HumanKinetics.com**.